Changing Human Behaviour to Enhance Animal Welfare

Changing Human Behaviour to Enhance Animal Welfare

Edited by Rebecca Sommerville

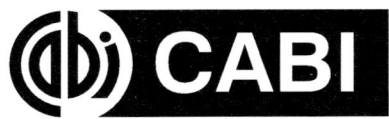

CABI is a trading name of CAB International

CABI
Nosworthy Way
Wallingford
Oxfordshire OX10 8DE
UK

Tel: +44 (0)1491 832111
Fax: +44 (0)1491 833508
E-mail: info@cabi.org
Website: www.cabi.org

CABI
WeWork
One Lincoln Street
24th Floor
Boston, MA 02111
USA

Tel: +1 (617)682-9015
E-mail: cabi-nao@cabi.org

© CAB International 2021. All rights reserved. No part of this publication may be reproduced in any form or by any means, electronically, mechanically, by photocopying, recording or otherwise, without the prior permission of the copyright owners.

A catalogue record for this book is available from the British Library, London, UK.

References to Internet websites (URLs) were accurate at the time of writing.

ISBN-13: 9781789247237 (paperback)
      9781789247244 (ePDF)
      9781789247251 (ePub)

DOI: 10.1079/9781789247237.0000

Commissioning Editor: Caroline Makepeace
Editorial Assistant: Lauren Davies
Production Editor: Marta Patiño

Typeset by SPi, Pondicherry, India
Printed and bound in the UK by Severn, Gloucester

Contents

Foreword   vii
Preface   ix
About the Contributors   xi

Part I.   Enhancing Animal Welfare – a Profession with Human
          Engagement at Its Centre

1. **The Need for Recognition of Practical Animal Welfare
    as a Profession**   1
    Rebecca Sommerville

2. **Animal Welfare: The Human Element**   20
    Suzanne Rogers and Jo White

3. **From Stakeholder Education to Engagement, Using Strategies
    from Social Science**   35
    Beth Ventura and Erica Hogstad Fjæran

4. **It Takes a Village: Community Engagement for Sustainable
    Animal Welfare**   48
    Melissa Liszewski

5. **Educating the Animal Welfare Practitioners of the Future**   65
    Cathy Dwyer, Heather Bacon, Tamsin Coombs and Fritha Langford

Part II: Enhancing Animal Welfare in Practice Worldwide

6. **Moving an Industry: Protecting Farm Animals with
    Science-based Advocacy**   82
    Sara Shields

7. **Applying the Science of Animal Welfare to Build More
    Responsible Food Supply Chains: Reflections from a
    Corporate Sustainability Professional**   97
    Priya Motupalli

8.	**Farm Animal Welfare in the Nigerian Context**	**113**
	Mabel Aworh-Ajumobi	
9.	**Protecting Animals in India: A Government Perspective through History to the Present Day**	**125**
	Vijay Pal Singh and Sujoy Khanna	
10.	**The Animals Powering the World: Promoting Working Animal Welfare in Resource-poor Contexts**	**141**
	Ashleigh F. Brown	
11.	**Strengthening Existing Healthcare Systems for Sustainable Animal Welfare**	**161**
	Shereene Williams and Laura Skippen	

Index   **179**

Foreword

The emphasis of this book is to work directly with the people who care for or use animals, to improve animal welfare. In my writings, I have often emphasized that the skills of stock people are not fully appreciated or acknowledged. On large corporate farms, the upper managers will often buy some fancy new technology instead of investing in the people who work with the animals. A major problem on some large farms run by distant corporate managers is that stock people are often overworked, underpaid and their skills are not fully acknowledged. On these farms, improvements in animal welfare will usually require upper-level management to fully support making changes. A large portion of my earlier animal welfare work was consulting with the upper-level managers of large meat buyers to train them to audit and monitor their farm suppliers. When I was first hired to do this work in the late 1990s, I brought upper-level corporate managers on their first trips to farms and slaughter plants. When they saw animals suffering, animal welfare was no longer an abstraction to be delegated to the legal or public relations department. Their eyes opened up and they had to do something about it. This approach was very effective for improving animal welfare in supply chains operated by managers who became motivated to improve animal welfare. Pressure from meat-buying consumers was another major motivator for many companies with highly visible brand names to eliminate poor practices. Unfortunately, there are still some major animal product supply chains that allow poor practices to continue because their customers are not concerned about animal welfare. In the egg industry, shell eggs with brand names are moving to cage-free, but the 'hidden' eggs going into bread or pastries are more likely to be in poorly monitored supply chains.

Changing Human Behaviour to Enhance Animal Welfare covers ways to improve welfare in situations where there is no large corporate buyer to enforce standards. Many of the chapters in the book cover working equids or village dogs. This requires a totally different approach compared to working with corporate supply managers. Many of the chapters describe successful work in low-income areas of countries such as Pakistan, Nigeria, India or Ethiopia.

In these situations, a working horse or donkey is essential for an individual's livelihood. To bring about improvements requires working within the community and strengthening existing networks for veterinary care. One example was educating local pharmacies about better veterinary treatments. Another approach was showing people that simple care practices would enable their horse or donkey to have a longer, more productive life. Some examples that are easy to implement are improvements in harnesses, using a spoon to clean hooves, making a curry comb out of bottle caps nailed to a board and providing more water. To motivate change requires working with local communities and acknowledging their contributions to a programme. Improvements need to come from within the community. A programme may fail if local people feel that their input is not being respected. One non-governmental organization (NGO) found this approach was more effective than providing free veterinary care. The emphasis is on working with the community rather than inspecting it. Priya Motupalli, the author of Chapter 7, states that the goal is 'progress over perfection'. I completely agree with this concept. Some of my work with large corporate meat buyers has been criticized because the animal-based outcome measures did not require perfection. There was a certain allowance for error. People who work in the field know that high standards can be attained but perfection is impossible.

Changing Human Behaviour to Enhance Animal Welfare is essential reading for people who are working to improve animal welfare in the local animals in a low-income area or developing country. It will also be helpful for people working in zoos or animal shelters. It is aimed at readers who are working directly with the people who care for the animals.

Temple Grandin
Department of Animal Science
Colorado State University

Preface

In recent years, the link between human behaviour change and animal welfare has increasingly been recognized. As the science of animal welfare grew, the focus was on the animal – how did they behave, what did they need and how could their welfare needs be met to avoid suffering and allow them to enjoy a good life? But these knowledge gains have not always translated into improvements to animals in practice with the expected impact. Highly industrialized agriculture has continued to spread, using systems that keep animals in confinement and prevent them from behaving naturally. Extreme breeding for aesthetic features continues to threaten the welfare of companion animals, whilst captive wildlife is still kept in unthinkable conditions for entertainment.

Working in international animal protection, I have witnessed a spectrum of welfare issues from farmed rabbits in barren cages in Europe, to donkeys and mules carrying heavy loads in brick kilns in South Asia, to rehabilitating rescue dogs in the UK. I have learnt that you have to work with the people closest to the animals, and positively influence their behaviour, to affect change. Whilst traditional campaigns have their place, often a complex dialogue and carefully selected methods of influence are required to create long-term, sustainable change. This goes beyond the powers of individual people, which is why systemic change is a key feature of this book. Animal owners and users can only change their behaviour within the confines of the system they live and work in – the industry or institution. As this book will show, the collective impact of professionals engaging in dialogue, building trust and working from the inside is beginning to fundamentally shift the way humans interact with animals.

Animal welfare research can be too far removed from the practical situation to be useful, but professionals finding, studying and applying the research specifically with the stakeholders they have built relationships with can lead to change. These professionals do exist and I have been fortunate enough to meet many of them around the world, several of whom have contributed to this book. The book was inspired by my work with international non-governmental organizations (NGOs). With a background in animal welfare science, I was recruited to translate the science into a digestible format for the NGOs to use. They wanted to make evidence-based arguments for change to their stakeholders, the animal owners and users. I came to recognize the gap between animal welfare science and its implementation into practice.

Unfortunately the work of these animal welfare professionals can be undervalued, because typically they are not high-profile, or senior leaders of universities, charities and businesses. Nor are they widely recognized as a unified profession – 'animal welfare practitioner' is not an existing role. This lack of recognition led me to take up a role as development officer for the International Society for Applied Ethology (ISAE), where I supported animal welfare and behaviour professionals in developing regions across Asia, Africa, eastern Europe and Latin America. I saw that they could make a difference to the welfare of animals in their country with access to the right professional training, experience and support.

This book discusses worldwide animal welfare issues, from professionals who live and work in low-, medium- and high-income countries (Fig. 0.1). Where they are represented by an international organization, voices from the field of the animal welfare practitioners working on the ground are heard through case studies. The book shares experiences from those who use the principles of animal welfare science and human behaviour change to influence the behaviour of animal owners and users. It will share how they make change happen in practice, including guidance and tips for others on how to translate the principles into real animal welfare impacts. My hope is that this book will serve as a stepping stone to recognizing animal welfare practitioners for the change they bring about, as their own indispensable profession.

Rebecca Sommerville
Editor

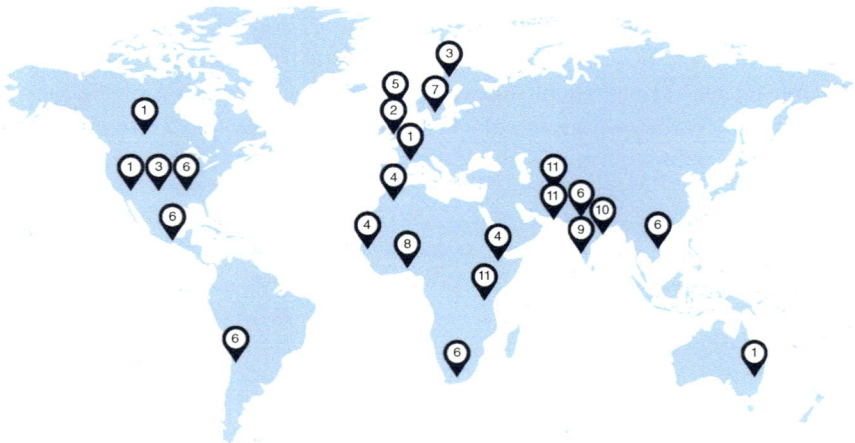

Fig. 0.1. A map highlighting the worldwide coverage of the book's animal welfare content. Each pin marks a country where the authors are based, have discussed projects or shared case studies from, with the chapter number inside the pin. They include the UK (Chapters 1, 2, 4, 5, 10, 11), France (1), Norway (3), Sweden (7), Canada (1), USA (1, 3, 6), Nigeria (8), Ethiopia (4, 10), Senegal (4), Morocco (4), Kenya (11), South Africa (6), India (6, 9, 10), Afghanistan (11), Pakistan (10, 11), Vietnam (6), Mexico (6), Chile (6) and Australia (1).

About the Contributors

Editor and Chapter 1

Rebecca Sommerville, Behaviour by Becca, London, UK. Email: behaviourbybecca@gmail.com

Rebecca Sommerville is a certificated clinical animal behaviourist and animal welfare scientist. She completed an MSc in applied animal behaviour and animal welfare at the University of Edinburgh and a BSc in animal behaviour at the University of Sheffield. Rebecca has worked as a post-adoption support behaviourist for Dogs Trust; a global animal welfare advisor for Brooke – Action for Working Horses and Donkeys; and a food business researcher for Compassion in World Farming. These roles involved working on human behaviour change with stakeholders from international food companies through to individual animal owners. Rebecca is a charity trustee of The Humane League UK and was formerly development officer for the International Society for Applied Ethology, promoting animal behaviour and welfare professionals in developing regions. She now supports dog owners and veterinarians through her business Behaviour by Becca, specializing in the rehabilitation of ex-racing greyhounds and rescue dogs.

Chapter 2

Suzanne Rogers, Human Behaviour Change for Animals CIC, UK. Email: suz@hbcforanimals.com

Jo White, Human Behaviour Change for Animals CIC, UK. Email: jo@hbcforanimals.com

Suzanne and Jo share a passion for animals and a fascination for what makes the human animal tick. Prior to joining forces to found Human Behaviour Change for Animals CIC, both had backgrounds in animal welfare and were working as consultants. They established Human Behaviour Change for Animals after recognizing that insight about how and why people behave the way they do could provide solutions to challenging issues that affect animals. After all, people interact with animals every day – by owning pets or farming animals, or through the choices we make about the food we eat or the clothes we wear. Between them, their knowledge, experience and qualifications cover animal behaviour, welfare and management; running international animal welfare programmes; and an MSc in (human) behaviour change. Fascinated by how to deliver positive change, they are committed to making a lasting difference by supporting others to use the principles and practice behind behaviour change.

Chapter 3

Beth Ventura, Department of Animal Science, University of Minnesota, St. Paul, Minnesota, USA. Email: bventura@umn.edu
Erica Hogstad Fjæran, Foreningen Norske Etologer (Association of Norwegian Ethologists), Steinkjer, Norway. Email: ericahf@gmail.com
Beth Ventura holds a PhD in applied animal biology/welfare from the University of British Columbia, Canada. As an animal welfare scientist and associate teaching professor at the University of Minnesota in the USA, she teaches courses on applied ethology and welfare to hundreds of undergraduate and postgraduate students. Her research interests span a range of topics, including the application of methods from the social sciences to address the human-level barriers preventing welfare improvements for animals. Erica Hogstad Fjæran earned her MSc in animal science and ethology from the Norwegian University of Life Sciences, including exchange and field work experience from Canada and Tanzania. Having worked in agricultural organizations and municipal management she strives to apply ethology in compliance with a One Welfare scope. Erica also has continued education in animal-assisted interventions, chairs the Norwegian Ethology Association, and works to communicate and emphasize scientific behaviour knowledge through freelance writing.

Chapter 4

Melissa Liszewski, International Fund for Animal Welfare (IFAW), London, UK. Email: mliszewski@ifaw.org
Melissa Liszewski leads the global Community Engagement Program at IFAW, an animal welfare and conservation organization working in over 40 countries, where she focuses on engaging communities in animal rescue, disaster risk reduction, mitigating human–wildlife conflict, combatting illegal wildlife trade and protecting vital habitats. She is a trustee for the Society for the Protection of Animals Abroad (SPANA), a working animal charity providing treatment, training and teaching around the world. Melissa previously led the global Community Development team at Brooke, an international organization

working to improve the lives of working equids and their communities. Her background is in animal science (behaviour and welfare), international development and social science, and she has worked on a range of other initiatives around the world since 2005 including farm animal policy in the USA, animal welfare education assessment in Austria, on-farm welfare assessment in Costa Rica, gibbon rescue in Thailand and working horse welfare in Brazil.

Chapter 5

Cathy Dwyer, The Royal (Dick) School of Veterinary Studies, University of Edinburgh, UK. Scotland's Rural College (SRUC), Edinburgh, UK. Email: cathy.dwyer@ed.ac.uk
Heather Bacon, The Royal (Dick) School of Veterinary Studies, University of Edinburgh, UK. Email: heather.bacon@ed.ac.uk
Tamsin Coombs, SRUC, Edinburgh, UK. Email: tamsin.coombs@sruc.ac.uk
Fritha Langford, SRUC, Edinburgh, UK. Email: fritha.langford@sruc.ac.uk
The University of Edinburgh, with SRUC, has been involved in animal welfare education since 1990 when the MSc course in applied animal behaviour and welfare began. Since 2011 the Jeanne Marchig International Centre for Animal Welfare Education (JMICAWE) has been part of the Royal (Dick) School of Veterinary Studies, with a global mission to provide education in animal welfare for veterinarians. In addition, a new online MSc programme in international animal welfare, ethics and law began in 2013. Professor Cathy Dwyer is the current director of JMICAWE, and teaches on both the MSc programmes as well as to undergraduate students. Dr Bacon is a veterinarian and part of JMICAWE where she leads the development of veterinary education in animal welfare. Drs Fritha Langford and Tamsin Coombs are the current programme directors of the two MSc programmes in animal welfare at the Royal (Dick) School of Veterinary Studies.

Chapter 6

Sara Shields, Humane Society International (HSI), Washington, USA. Email: sshields@hsi.org
Dr Sara Shields earned her BSc in zoology from Colorado State University and her PhD from the University of California, Davis in animal behavior in 2004, where she completed her doctoral research on the behaviour of broiler chickens. She taught animal welfare classes and did postdoctoral research on laying hen behaviour and nutrition at the University of Nebraska, Lincoln. She is currently the director of Farm Animal Welfare Science at HSI and has been working for HSI and the Humane Society of the United States for 14 years. She specializes in the welfare of farm animals and provides scientific and technical information to government, food retailers, universities, producers, law

enforcement, standard-setting bodies and advocacy organizations. She is a published author of several original research articles, reviews and organizational white papers. She served as a US delegate to the International Organization for Standardization (ISO) TC34 Working Group on Animal Welfare. She is past-chair of the International Coalition for Animal Welfare (ICFAW), the official NGO body recognized by the World Organisation for Animal Health (OIE). She is currently a board member of Global Animal Partnership, a farm animal standard-setting and certification programme.

Chapter 7

Priya Motupalli, IKEA Food, Malmö, Sweden. Email: priya.motupalli@inter.ikea.com

Dr Priya Motupalli currently leads on the development of the sustainable sourcing agenda for the animal products in the IKEA Food range. Her unique background spans three sectors, multiple geographies and multiple species, giving her a holistic outlook connected to animal welfare in food supply chains. Prior to working with IKEA Food she completed a PhD focusing on the impact of choice on dairy cattle welfare and production. She then moved into the non-profit sector supporting large food businesses to improve animal welfare at the farm level via technical expertise and strategy development. Her research and insights have been featured in multiple mediums both academic and popular, including the *Journal of Animal Science, Scientific American, Triple Pundit,* and NPR's *Tell Me Something I Don't Know*. She is also an invited speaker globally on the intersection of business and animal welfare.

Chapter 8

Mabel Aworh-Ajumobi, Department of Veterinary and Pest Control Services, Federal Ministry of Agriculture and Rural Development, Abuja, Nigeria. Email: mabelaworh@yahoo.com

Dr Mabel Aworh-Ajumobi is an epidemiologist with over a decade of experience in veterinary epidemiology, public health, global health, food safety, research and leadership, including as head of the Animal Welfare Unit of the Department of Veterinary Services, Federal Ministry of Agriculture and Rural Development, Abuja, Nigeria. She received her Doctor of Veterinary Medicine degree and Master's in public health (field epidemiology) in Nigeria. Dr Aworh-Ajumobi has conducted research focused on One Health issues, led research and survey teams, and published in peer-reviewed journals. She is a two-time recipient of the International Society for Applied Ethology (ISAE) Developing Countries Congress Attendance Fellowship and is the ISAE country liaison for Nigeria. She is the OIE national focal point for animal welfare in Nigeria. Her current research as a Fleming fund fellow is on drug-resistant *E. coli* in beef cattle and slaughterhouse workers.

Chapter 9

Vijay Pal Singh, Council of Scientific and Industrial Research - Institute of Genomics and Integrative Biology. Email: vp.singh@igib.in

Sujoy Khanna, Lala Lajpat Rai University of Veterinary and Animal Sciences (LUVAS), Hisar, India. Email: joykhanna20@gmail.com

Vijay Pal Singh is a veterinary graduate with a PhD in biotechnology. As a veterinarian and assistant professor of biological sciences at the Academy of Scientific and Innovative Research, he teaches laboratory animal welfare in India and abroad. He is the Indian country liaison for the International Society of Applied Ethology, part of the Animal Welfare Focus group of the World Veterinary Association and an ad hoc consultant for the American Association for Accreditation of Laboratory Animal Care. Sujoy Khanna is a veterinarian with a doctorate in livestock production management. He is an assistant professor teaching scientific, ethical and other dimensions of animal welfare and livestock production. He wrote a book entitled *Gaushala* with Mrs. Maneka Sanjay Gandhi, on transforming cattle shelters in India. This aroused considerable interest towards animal welfare activities and he began working at a grassroots village level to bring about improvements in farm animal welfare.

Chapter 10

Ashleigh F. Brown, international animal behaviour and welfare scientist. Email: ashleighfionabrown@gmail.com

With a background in applied ethology, animal welfare science, education and development management, Ashleigh currently works in a scientific advisory capacity for international charity, Brooke Action for Working Horses and Donkeys, and seconded to the World Bank for an equine welfare project. She has been a trustee for wildlife and conservation charities (Friends of Inti Wara Yassi and League Against Cruel Sports); a member of the International Society for Applied Ethology, Association for the Study of Animal Behaviour, Universities' Federation for Animal Welfare and International Society for Equitation Science; and a contributing writer for the Global Animal Network. Ashleigh is part of TEDxLondon's leadership team, a lay advisor for the Royal College of Surgeons of Edinburgh and the Academy of Medical Royal Colleges, and an academic and career mentor for young people. Having worked or travelled in almost 80 countries, Ashleigh has particular interests in the inter-relationship between animal welfare and international development, and in animal welfare education worldwide. When not globetrotting, she can be found enjoying city life in London or recharging back home in Scotland.

Chapter 11

Shereene Williams, Brooke Action for Working Horses and Donkeys, London, UK. Email: shereene.williams@thebrooke.org

Laura Skippen, Brooke Action for Working Horses and Donkeys, London, UK. Email: laura.skippen@thebrooke.org

Shereene qualified as a veterinary surgeon in 2011 from Nottingham Vet School, UK. She started her career at the equine welfare organization Redwings and worked alongside the RSPCA at the famous Appleby Horse Fair. Shereene joined Brooke Action for Working Horses and Donkeys as a global animal health advisor in 2016. Shereene focuses on improving access to essential medicines, One Health and working to professionalize farriery in low- to middle-income countries. Laura qualified as a vet in 2005 from the Royal Veterinary College and worked in mixed and equine practice in the UK. Having joined Brooke Action for Working Horses and Donkeys in 2012, she supports animal health practitioners to provide high-quality healthcare to improve the lives of working animals. Having gaining qualifications in veterinary education, Laura works with veterinary training institutions in low- and middle-income countries to include animal welfare and practical clinical skills within their curricula.

The Need for Recognition of Practical Animal Welfare as a Profession

1

Rebecca Sommerville
Behaviour by Becca, London, UK

1.1 Introduction

The welfare of animals is intricately linked with human wellbeing and the environment, a concept known as 'One Welfare' (García Pinillos, 2018). Today the biomass of humans and domestic livestock on the planet outweighs that of all vertebrate wildlife (except fishes), mainly comprising chickens, cows and pigs (Bar-On *et al.*, 2018). With this vast number of animals managed by, or interacting with, humans we need to engage with people to improve the animals' welfare – to prevent suffering and to ensure a good quality of life. Animal welfare science provides evidence about what animals need and want. There are several books about what animal welfare means (e.g. Grandin, 2015; Appleby *et al.*, 2018) and why it matters (McMillan, 2020), but few describe how to translate this into everyday actions and who makes this change happen. This gap between science and existing practices can be a challenge to bridge.

There are well-established professions in veterinary health, animal welfare science, clinical behaviour and applied animal behaviour, yet there is no field of 'practical animal welfare'. There isn't a widely recognized role of an 'animal welfare practitioner' who translates animal welfare principles into practice. There is a need to recognize this distinct profession of individuals who work closely with the animals and their owners, carers, communities or users to improve animal welfare. Such professionals already exist and are based at non-governmental organizations (NGOs), charities, governments, industries and universities, with roles as animal welfare advisors, researchers, welfare assessors or veterinarians with additional animal welfare expertise.

This book sets out to give an insight into these professionals' lives, with a chapter each to share their view and ways of working, while offering practical guidance to others who want to improve animal welfare. It highlights the need for recognition of the field of 'practical animal welfare'. The importance of human behaviour change to animal welfare is increasingly recognized and therefore is a core theme of this book. Legislation can be passed to outlaw practices that lead to poor welfare, but the practice will continue if there is no enforcement, or if legislators have little knowledge of the field conditions (Grandin, 2015). Behaviour change of individuals isn't enough alone, however, to create lasting animal welfare improvements. Therefore, how to make systemic changes to whole institutions and industries is another theme of this book.

The authors featured and their work have a truly international focus, because while the field of animal welfare science began in Europe, North America and Australasia, it is growing across Asia, Africa and Latin America, as research groups are established, international and grassroots NGOs undertake projects and governments implement guidelines, such as from the World Organisation for Animal Health (OIE). This book suggests resources to use, describes case studies, and discusses the barriers, solutions and future directions in the field of practical animal welfare. The book aims to help budding animal welfare practitioners to get involved and for existing practitioners to get the recognition they deserve for their often 'behind the scenes' work.

- Part I 'Enhancing Animal Welfare – a Profession with Human Engagement at Its Centre', describes the scientific theories and principles that underpin human behaviour and systemic change to enhance animal welfare. There are examples from companion animals (Chapters 2 and 5), farm animals (Chapters 3 and 5) and wildlife (Chapter 4).
- Part II 'Enhancing Animal Welfare in Practice Worldwide' describes the realities in practice, hearing the voices of animal welfare practitioners in different sectors describe how they work. There are examples from farm animals (Chapters 6–9), wildlife (Chapters 9 and 10) and working equids (Chapters 10 and 11).

1.2 What Is Animal Welfare?

Animal welfare comprises an animal's physical functioning to survive (Fraser and Broom, 1990), their ability to express natural behaviour (Rollin, 1992) and their emotional state (Duncan, 1996) (see Chapter 3). When their survival needs are met and they can express rewarding behaviours, animals thrive and enjoy good welfare. Emotional states promote survival by prompting an animal to behave in a certain way. Negative emotional states from sensations inside the body include: hunger, thirst, pain, breathlessness, nausea, dizziness, debility, weakness and sickness. Those from perceiving the environment include: fear, anxiety, frustration, panic, vigilance, boredom, depression, loneliness and helplessness (Mellor and Beausoleil, 2020).

By reducing negative experiences, welfare can only be negative or neutral; it's not possible to avoid all negative states because some are essential for survival. To enhance welfare, negative experiences should be minimized to a tolerable level that still allows life-sustaining behaviours, such as eating, drinking, resting, ceasing activity when unwell and seeking warmth or shade (Mellor and Beausoleil, 2020). In order to avoid suffering, negative states should not be permitted to become chronic, long-term experiences. Positive emotional states are caused by the body's experience, or anticipation of rewards. Positive emotional states include: pleasure, comfort, interest and a sense of control.

Since their origin, the five freedoms of animal welfare (Brambell, 1965) have contributed to laws and policies worldwide, however there is increasing recognition that they don't go far enough (Mellor and Beausoleil, 2020). The focus on 'freedom from' a negative state prevents efforts towards positive animal welfare, which are essential for an animal to thrive and feel good, beyond just surviving (Boissy *et al.*, 2007). The five domains of welfare are a useful concept that build on the five freedoms and now take into account the potential positive and negative influences of human behaviour on animal welfare (Mellor *et al.*, 2020). The domains have taken longer to be taken up into global practice. This is changing because they are a useful framework to assess all of the components of animal welfare. Undertaking welfare assessment is needed to understand the current state of the animals' conditions, to provide objective evidence and a baseline to monitor progress against for the individual or group.

The provisions of animal welfare, from the Five Domains Model (Mellor, 2016; Mellor *et al.*, 2020) are:

1. Good nutrition: provide ready access to fresh water and a diet to maintain full health and vigour.
2. Good environment: provide shade/shelter or suitable housing, good air quality and comfortable resting areas.
3. Good health: prevent or rapidly diagnose and treat disease and injury, and foster good muscle tone, posture and cardiorespiratory function.
4. Behavioural interaction: provide positive interactions with the environment, other animals and humans.
5. Positive mental experiences: provide safe, congenial and species-appropriate opportunities to have pleasurable experiences.

Figure 1.1 is an example of how the domains can be used in practice as an education tool with an animal owner, community, NGO, government or industry staff member who does not have an animal welfare science background. Combining welfare measures into a single score is not recommended, because weighing one score against another is subjective and higher scores in one area can mask poor welfare measures that are unacceptable in another area (Grandin, 2015). A more detailed tool and training of assessors is required for a full welfare assessment. Here are some example questions to consider with your stakeholder while using this summary:

- How many positive vs negative states do the animal/s have?
- Which of these apply to your animals' species-specific behaviour?
- How long do their positive and negative experiences last for?
- What are the frequency, intensity and severity of their experiences?
- Are some experiences better or worse than others?

ANIMAL WELFARE DOMAINS
A VISUAL SUMMARY

PROVISIONS: WHAT YOU GIVE TO THE ANIMAL		MENTAL STATES: HOW THE ANIMAL FEELS (EXAMPLES)	
		YES POSITIVE	**NO** NEGATIVE
1. NUTRITION			
• Is there enough food?		• Pleasure	• Hunger
• Is there enough water?		• Quenched	• Thirst
• Is there enough food variety?		• Pleasure	• Malaise
• Is there no overeating?		• Satiated	• Bloated
• Is there no force-feeding?		• Comfort	• Pain
2. ENVIRONMENT		**YES**	**NO**
• Is the temperature tolerable?		• Comfort	• Chilled
• Is the floor substrate suitable?		• Comfort	• Overheated
• Is there space for free movement?		• Comfort	• Irritation
• Is the air fresh?		• Comfort	• Breathless
• Are the odours, light & noise tolerable?		• Comfort	• Anxious
3. HEALTH		**YES**	**NO**
• Is there no disease?		• Comfort	• Sick
• Is there no injury?		• Comfort	• Pain
• Can they function normally?		• Comfort	• Weak
• Are they physically fit?		• Functioning	• Debilitated
• Are they lean and not obese?		• Vitality	• Breathless
5. BEHAVIOURAL INTERACTIONS		**YES**	**NO**
• Is the environment varied or novel?		• Interested	• Bored
• Are there engaging choices available?		• In control	• Anger
• Can they forage, hunt, or do substitutes?		• Focused	• Frustration
• Can they form social bonds, or hide away?		• Affectionate	• Lonely
• How are their interactions with humans?		• Secure	• Fear

= OVERALL WELFARE STATUS

Fig. 1.1. A summary of the Five Domains Model. (Derived from Mellor and Beausoleil, 2020 and Mellor *et al.*, 2020.)

1.3 How Should Animal Welfare Practitioners Be Trained?

Formal training in animal welfare is required to become an animal welfare practitioner; it is not sufficient to have a degree in veterinary health or animal behaviour because the role requires an in-depth understanding of an animal's mental wellbeing, not just physical health, the components of welfare and how to assess these. There are many different routes to become an animal welfare practitioner and to continue lifelong learning, including:

- undergraduate degrees;
- postgraduate MSc/PhD;
- short courses;
- association memberships;
- work shadowing, volunteering, internships;
- on-the-job training, e.g. in an NGO, government or industry role;
- practical experience 'in the field', e.g. as a welfare assessor; and
- conference or workshop attendance.

In this book, the authors share their different routes to becoming an animal welfare practitioner, as they work in a wide variety of roles with different animal species. They include individuals working for an NGO (Chapters 1, 2, 4, 6, 10 and 11), university (Chapter 3), industry (Chapter 7) and government

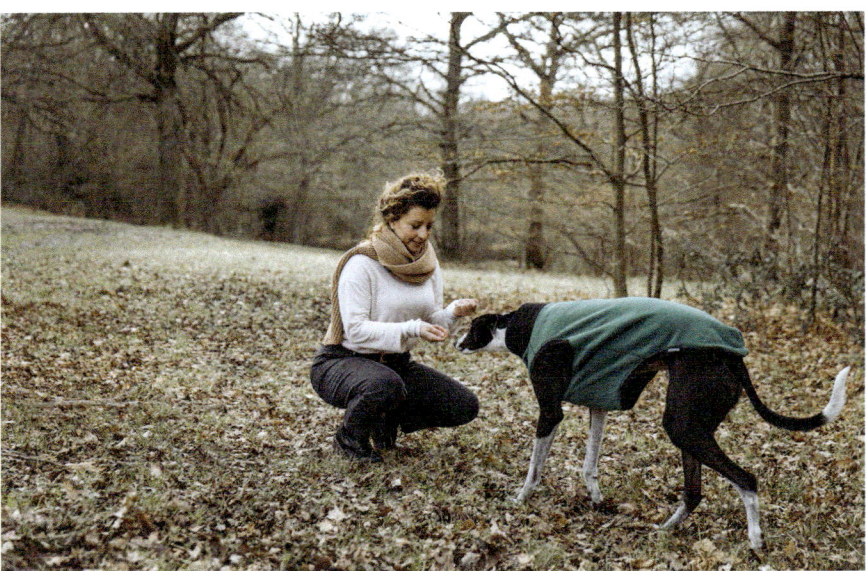

Fig. 1.2. As an animal welfare practitioner, author Rebecca uses her training in animal welfare and clinical behaviour to rehabilitate ex-racing greyhounds. (© Freya Dowson.)

(Chapters 8 and 9). Chapter 5 describes routes to obtaining the education and Chapter 10 the practical field experience required to become a practitioner.

1.4 How Do Practitioners Engage People in Animal Welfare?

The two overarching methods leading to animal welfare progress are individual human behaviour change and institutional systemic change. The principles of behaviour change are described in Chapters 2, 3 and 4. Examples of the variety of approaches used to change human behaviour or the system are given in Table 1.1. This table demonstrates that there is no single right way to create change, there are many approaches, and which approach is most suitable depends on the stakeholders, what they will be receptive to and the surrounding conditions. Monitoring and evaluating the effectiveness of the chosen approach during and after a project is essential.

1.5 Looking to the Future of the Field

This book and chapter feature case studies from animal welfare practitioners working with farm, research, wildlife and companion animals, with a wide diversity of approaches. The importance of the field of applying animal welfare to real-life practice shouldn't be undervalued and it is hoped that animal welfare institutions, NGOs, governments and veterinary departments will recognize and strengthen the profession of practical animal welfare. A promising sign is the increase in the study, groups and conferences focusing on human behaviour change. In turn these talented professionals will use their expertise and experience to improve the quality of life of animals worldwide, by working closely with their owners and users and influencing positive change in the systems and institutions overarching these.

Case Study 1: Using Welfare Science to Assess the Welfare of Captive Whales and Dolphins

Dr Isabella Clegg
Animal Welfare Expertise, Sydney, Australia
www.animalwelfareexpertise.com (accessed 30 March 2021)

Whales and dolphins, otherwise known as 'cetaceans', are kept in zoos and aquariums globally, but intense public debate surrounds this practice in many countries. Two critical questions define people's ethical positions: 'Do cetaceans have good or poor welfare in captivity?' and 'What is the purpose of them being there?'. Fortunately, welfare science is finally starting to provide objective evidence for the first question. This is the subject of her work: Dr Clegg conducts welfare assessments of captive cetaceans and other animals in order to improve the animals' welfare and provide the public with unbiased information (Fig. 1.3).

Continued

Case Study 1: Continued.

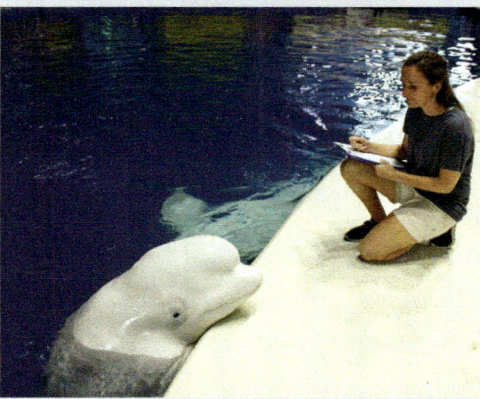

Fig. 1.3. Dr Isabella Clegg assessing the welfare of a captive Beluga whale.

Dr Clegg's approach to welfare assessment is collaborative and not punitive: she works *with* the facilities as opposed to 'inspecting' them. This allows her to collect more meaningful data on the animals and operations, and effectively suggest and implement improvements. Since zoo animal welfare is a new field there were very few jobs available when she finished her PhD (on dolphin welfare), so she founded the consultancy Animal Welfare Expertise (AWE). AWE's guiding principle is to bridge the gap between academia and industry by translating welfare science approaches to animal facilities.

Through AWE, Dr Clegg has been involved in a wide variety of cetacean welfare projects. She has applied the Cetacean Welfare ('C-Well©') Assessment (Clegg *et al.*, 2015) to many captive cetacean groups. One of the main recommendations for facilities is to improve their enrichment programmes, particularly to increase the cognitive challenges available to cetaceans when they are not being trained to alleviate boredom. To this end, she established a platform called IdeaBox to facilitate the sharing of innovative ideas for cetacean enrichment. Dr Clegg has assessed the welfare of cetaceans moved to 'sanctuaries' – large sea pens where breeding and public interactions are prohibited. She and her co-authors are starting to apply findings on emotional states from captive research to wild cetacean conservation efforts. Dr Clegg is very grateful to all facility and sanctuary directors for embracing welfare assessments so far: collecting objective data is the only way to discover which settings and practices actually improve cetacean welfare.

Approaches used for individual or systemic change

- research and industry collaboration;
- welfare assessment tools; and
- business engagement and industry standards.

Case Study 2: Making Progress Through Engagement and Campaigning

Vicky Bond
Managing Director, The Humane League, Brighton, UK

By the end of studying for her veterinary degree, Vicky knew she wanted to end the suffering of animals raised for food. Vicky's first advocacy job was at Compassion in World Farming, where she started in research, before moving to work with food businesses on their farms and in slaughterhouses to improve welfare.

Since 2017 Vicky has led the The Humane League (THL) after they started operating in the UK in 2016, becoming a charity in 2018. Originating in the USA, THL brought a new way to persuade companies to improve welfare standards in their supply chains. They work collaboratively with food businesses when they are willing to engage, or run public campaigns to raise awareness of poor welfare conditions, when they aren't. This successful method has moved some of the largest companies in the world to commit to higher welfare standards, including KFC (Levitt, 2020), Sodexo and Tesco, helping millions of animals every year.

Through the 'Better Chicken Commitment', an NGO initiative for broiler chickens, over 170 food companies have agreed to improve their stocking density, enrichment, slaughter and auditing, and to use a higher-welfare breed (Fig. 1.4).

In another example, THL had initial discussions with Noble Foods, the largest egg producer in the UK, to stop using cages in their supply chain. These were not fruitful because the company did not believe that consumers cared, so THL began a public campaign using articles in major media outlets. These highlighted the double standard of Noble Foods owning the free-range brand 'Happy Eggs' while keeping hens in cages for their other brands. Public support grew, with over 75,000 people signing a petition. An undercover investigation by another NGO Animal Equality revealing poor welfare conditions on their farms, combined with THL's demonstrations outside Noble Foods' offices, drew press attention. This was the final factor that led to Noble Foods committing to 100% cage-free eggs by 2025, benefiting over 4 million hens a year.

Approaches used for individual or systemic change

- campaigns;
- lobbying and advocacy; and
- business engagement and industry standards.

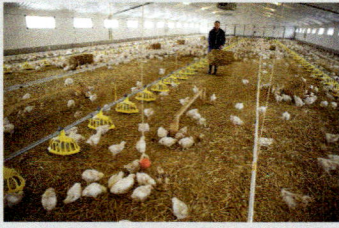

Fig. 1.4. A higher-welfare indoor system for broiler chickens with natural light, more space and enrichment. (© RSPCA Assured and Alexander Caminada, https://caminada.co.uk, accessed 30 March 2021.)

Case Study 3: Tickling Rats and Training Personnel for Improved Laboratory Animal Welfare

Dr Megan LaFollette
The North American 3Rs Collaborative

When laboratory rats are first handled, they can experience fear, stress and anxiety, which harms welfare and scientific results (Gärtner et al., 1980; Brudzynski and Ociepa, 1992; Morgan and Tromborg, 2007). These negative effects can be compounded by common procedures such as restraint, injection or blood draws (Balcombe et al. 2004). Fortunately, handling stress can be mitigated through the positive handling technique of rat tickling (Fig. 1.5). This interaction mimics aspects of rat rough-and-tumble play, increases positive affect and approach behaviour, and benefits handling (LaFollette et al., 2017).

Dr Megan LaFollette's MSc and PhD research projects focused on the practical application of rat tickling in the research laboratory. First, she conducted a systematic review on rat tickling to ensure that there truly was a strong scientific literature base to support its application (LaFollette et al., 2017). Then, she surveyed laboratory animal personnel to establish prevalence and barriers to use (LaFollette et al., 2019). After finding that common barriers were time, buy-in and lack of training, she set out to complete two projects to address those barriers. First, she conducted a study showing only 15 s of tickling for 3 days is effective (LaFollette et al., 2018). Second, she conducted a study in which she created an online rat tickling certificate that had extensive video/pictorial elements and addressed common difficulties with the technique (LaFollette et al., 2020). This project found that either online-only training or online and hands-on training was effective in improving implementation, knowledge, self-efficacy and familiarity with rat tickling.

Currently, Dr LaFollette is a 3Rs fellow for The North American 3Rs Collaborative, where she uses the knowledge she gained during her graduate studies to advance the education and science of refining, reducing and replacing the use of animals in research. For example, she creates easily digested webpages, newsletters and podcasts of best practices that address common barriers to use. In each, she focuses first on *why* the topic is important, then *what* to do and finally directly addresses common barriers, linking out to more detailed resources. Her efforts help translate welfare science into real-life practice.

Approaches used for individual or systemic change

- research and industry collaboration;
- education; and
- social marketing: print or TV media, websites, social media.

Continued

Case Study 3: Continued.

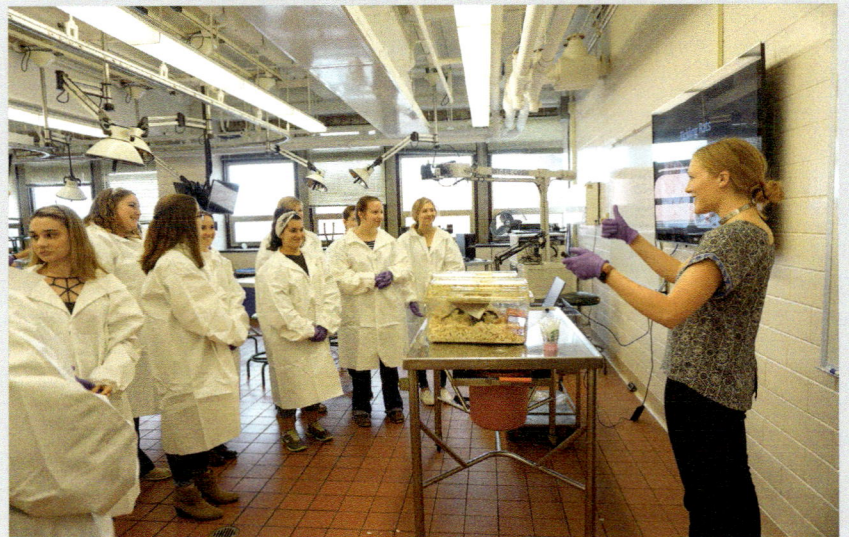

Fig. 1.5. Dr LaFollette running a workshop on rat tickling.

Case Study 4: The Five Domains Model Successfully Used in a Cruelty Case Involving a Choked Cat

Dr Rebecca Ledger
Langara College, Vancouver, Canada

The vast majority of animal cruelty prosecutions involve cases where there is clear physical evidence of abuse. Given that animals can suffer from affective states in the absence of physical harm, this has left many cases of animal abuse overlooked by the courts.

Since 2014 in Canada however, such cases have been successfully prosecuted by utilizing behavioural evidence of negative affect in a range of species, including dogs, rabbits, pigs and cats.

In June 2019, in R. vs Rodgers-Langille, the Cartmouth Provincial Court (Nova Scotia) found a 20-year-old man guilty of animal cruelty after the accused sent three short videos to his girlfriend of himself choking her cat, Oscar. Oscar survived and was immediately seized by the Nova Scotia Society for Prevention of Cruelty to Animals (SPCA). On physical examination, the veterinarian concluded that Oscar 'showed no obvious damage from being strangled'.

Expert witness Dr Rebecca Ledger applied the Five Domains Model to demonstrate Oscar had suffered from anxiety, fear, physical discomfort, pain, panic and breathlessness based on the conditions Oscar was subjected to, and his behavioural response.

Rodgers-Langille was sentenced to 150 days in jail, followed by 2 days' probation, and prohibited from owning any animal for 10 years.

Approaches used for behaviour or systemic change

- legislation, international standards and enforcement.

How to Change the Behaviour of Farmers and Food Businesses Rearing Rabbits

Rebecca Sommerville, Dr Tracey Jones and Jo Cooper
Compassion in World Farming (CIWF), Godalming, UK
www.compassioninfoodbusiness.com (accessed 30 March 2021)

1. Identify the problem

Rabbits are the second-most farmed species in Europe, after chickens, with more than 180 million rabbits slaughtered every year in the European Union (EU) (European Council, 2017). Most rabbits are reared in industrial caged systems and there is no species-specific legislation to protect their welfare. They are generally housed at high stocking densities, with restricted head height, in barren cages with wired flooring, which prevents them from expressing natural behaviours such as lying stretched out, rearing up on their hind legs, hopping and gnawing. Mortality rates are high owing to disease and high levels of antibiotics are routinely used. Breeding rabbits (does) are housed individually in wire cages that deny them social interaction.

2. Investigate solutions

In order to raise the baseline standards of welfare for rabbits, work needed to be done to encourage the industry to move their production to cage-free systems. Following Kaufland's 2013 Best Retailer Innovation Award and BreFood's 2014 Rabbit Innovation Award for cage-free meat rabbit production, CIWF's Food Business team undertook desk research and visited farms and slaughterhouses across Europe and China using a variety of cage-free housing systems in order to define key criteria for non-caged production.

A parallel investigation by CIWF's campaigns team revealed the poor conditions of rabbits housed in cages, which helped raise public support for change. A meta-analysis of the existing evidence, in collaboration with the Spanish research institute Neiker Tecnalia, was published (Sommerville *et al.*, 2017), and information sheets on rabbit welfare provided credible evidence to share with food businesses.

3. Apply your approach to behaviour change

The Food Business team's approach involved setting new standards for the industry and publicly recognizing those companies making positive changes. The Good Rabbit Award is a good example of driving change by bringing people on board with sound scientific and practical evidence and encouraging them to take ownership of the developments and solutions. The award recognizes companies making a commitment to use higher-welfare systems for does and meat rabbits (Fig. 1.6). The criteria for meat rabbits include: cage-free housing, no pen height restriction, comfortable flooring, enrichment, a dawn–dusk lighting schedule, natural light and no routine use of antibiotics. The criteria for does include: group housing (unless with their unweaned offspring, kits), measures to minimize aggression and nesting material.

4. Driving continuous improvement

Since the Good Rabbit Award was launched in 2015, the Food Business team has worked with a number of companies across Europe to help them introduce the new standards and, to date, over 8.4 million rabbits are set to benefit each year.

Continued

Continued.

To be commercially viable, companies need to bring consumers on the journey with them. One example is Eleveurs et Bien – a joint partnership between three major players that represent 60% of the French rabbit industry – CPLB Groupe Cavac, Terrena and Loeul & Piriot – who joined forces to launch a new housing system where the rabbits are reared in large pens which feature a burrow-style area, allowing them to hide and rest, as well as substrates and blocks to gnaw on, and much increased space availability. To meet the growing demands of the market for higher-welfare rabbit meat, they also launched their commercial brand Lapin & Bien in 2019.

While legislation is still lacking, the welfare of farmed rabbits is under the spotlight, as are caged farming systems. The European Food Safety Authority's report (AHAW *et al.*, 2020) concluded that the welfare of adult rabbits is lower in conventional cages than in other housing systems, the welfare of kits is highest in elevated pens and that organic systems are generally good, setting the scene for future change.

According to a poll (YouGov, 2020), 88% of people agreed that using cages in farming is cruel to animals and CIWF's groundbreaking European Citizens Initiative (ECI) recently inspired over 1.6 million people and 170 organizations across Europe to stand up and demand an end to using cages for farm animals.

Consumers have clearly spoken out against caged farming and, although further work is still required for cage-free doe production to become the norm, the commercial knowhow is there to allow for a successful transition to cage-free production for all rabbits in future.

Approaches used for individual or systemic change

- incentive schemes;
- business engagement and industry standards; and
- research and industry collaboration.

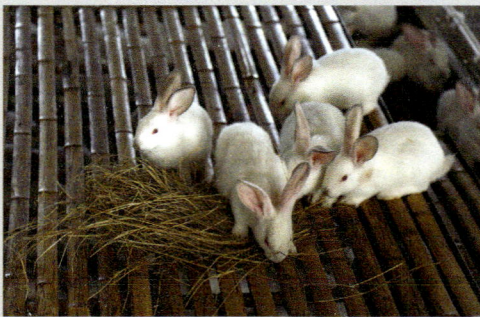

Fig. 1.6. A higher-welfare indoor system for growing rabbits, with more space, places to hide and enrichment.

1.6 Recommended Resources

- International Society for Applied Ethology, https://www.applied-ethology.org (accessed 30 March 2021).
- Human Behaviour Change for Animals, https://www.hbcforanimals.com (accessed 30 March 2021).
- World Organisation for Animal Health national animal welfare focal points, https://rr-europe.oie.int/en/the-oie-national-focal-points/animal-welfare-focal-points (accessed 30 March 2021).
- Commonwealth Veterinary Association and Congress, https://www.commonwealthvetassoc.com (accessed 30 March 2021).
- Universities Federation for Animal Welfare, https://www.ufaw.org.uk (accessed 30 March 2021).
- Animal Welfare Research Network, https://awrn.co.uk (accessed 30 March 2021).
- International Association of Animal Behaviour Consultants, https://m.iaabc.org (accessed 30 March 2021).
- International Companion Animal Management Coalition, https://www.icam-coalition.org (accessed 30 March 2021).
- International Conference on the Assessment of Animal Welfare at Farm and Group level, https://www.wafl2021.com (accessed 30 March 2021).
- Brazilian Ethology Society, www.etologiabrasil.org.br (accessed 30 March 2021).
- World Veterinary Association strategic focus group on animal welfare, http://worldvet.org/news.php?item=454 (accessed 30 March 2021).
- Africa Animal Welfare Conference, https://www.aawconference.org/index.php (accessed 30 March 2021).
- Global Animal Partnership, https://globalanimalpartnership.org (accessed 30 March 2021).
- Eurogroup for animals, https://www.eurogroupforanimals.org (accessed 30 March 2021).
- Open Philanthropy Project farm animal welfare, https://www.openphilanthropy.org/focus/us-policy/farm-animal-welfare (accessed 30 March 2021).
- Coalition of African Animal Welfare Organisations, https://www.caawo.org (accessed 30 March 2021).
- National Centre for the Replacement, Refinement and Reduction of Animals in Research, https://www.nc3rs.org.uk (accessed 30 March 2021).
- The Jeanne Marchig International Centre for Animal Welfare Education, https://www.ed.ac.uk/vet/jeanne-marchig-centre (accessed 30 March 2021).

Acknowledgements

The author is grateful to Dr Naomi Harvey for her feedback on this chapter, to Professor David Mellor for discussions about the conception of the chapter

Table 1.1. Approaches to enhancing animal welfare through individual human behaviour and institutional systemic change.

Approaches: How to create change	Benefits	Challenges	Example
Campaigns	Potential large-scale systemic change for millions of animals	Negative pressure campaigns prevent dialogue and can limit change if businesses don't want to respond to this pressure	Case Study 2
Lobbying and advocacy	Policy changes can affect animal groups or populations leading to long-term systemic change	Impact can be hard to assess if the policy is far removed from the animals	Case Study 2
Legislation, international standards and enforcement	Potential large-scale systemic change for millions of animals	Without enforcement no change is made. Legislation tends to involve the minimum standards to prevent suffering, rather than to provide positive welfare. International Animal Health standards (e.g. OIE) are voluntary, and require implementation at the field level	Chapters 8 and 9
Incentive schemes, assurance, certification	Positive incentives schemes have the potential for large-scale change. Certification by independent bodies typically involves a combination of welfare assessment and social marketing, such as labelling or media releases, which can encourage consumers to choose higher-welfare products	Commitments to award schemes by businesses are voluntary and require enforcement or they can be reneged on. Negative incentive schemes, such as inspections, auditing or using fines are a top-down approach, which may create bad feelings and dissuade owners from exceeding the minimum requirement to pass an inspection	Behaviour change box: rabbit farming

Approach	Description	Limitations	Reference
Business engagement and industry standards	For farmed animals, large food retailers (e.g. supermarkets), food service (e.g. restaurants, caterers), manufacturers, and small and medium enterprises (e.g. schools, university canteens) can set their own commitments, which can be quick to publish and require higher standards than legislation and involve standard operating procedures to meet them	Changes to supply chains take a long time and require consumer demand, and therefore may be reliant on feeling pressure to change from the other approaches listed here first. Food businesses offering cheap or fast food at the lower end of the price scale may not be interested, as their consumers are concerned with cost above welfare. If compliance to standards is focused on keeping records and filling out forms instead of monitoring, suffering can continue	Chapters 6, 7 and Case Study 4
Education	Formal education, such as teaching animal welfare at schools and universities leads to generational change. Informal education, such as farmers visiting other farms, or taking part in discussion groups led by NGOs leads to smaller-scale immediate changes	Change must be owned, stakeholders must believe in the required behaviours in order to carry them out	Chapter 5
Research and industry collaboration	University and industry or NGO collaborations encourage evidence-based practice. Recommendations that come from a credible independent source are more likely to be followed than those from an NGO perceived as having an agenda	Communication of results may be limited owing to business competition rules. The number of animals reached depends on research and industry funding available	Chapter 7 and Case Study 1

Continued

Table 1.1. Continued.

Approaches: How to create change	Benefits	Challenges	Example
Community groups, associations and representatives	Community groups and associations empower individuals to make change with a bottom-up approach that can be highly effective, as changes are owned, e.g. Participatory Rural Appraisal. 'Change agents' are motivated community representatives who receive training and can change practices in their community	The welfare changes made depend on the existing knowledge, attitudes and practice of the community, or the skills of an external facilitator to enable this. The number of animals reached is limited to the size of the community group and the scale of the project implementation across communities	Chapter 4
Alternative livelihoods	Long-term welfare changes can be made if practices that cause suffering are replaced, or the number of animals reduced. Owners or users have a route out of practising poor welfare, as they are supported to find a new livelihood	Schemes that are not fully participatory are likely to fail because the owner or user's livelihood is also part of their identity. The number of animals reached is likely to be on a small scale owing to the resources required	Chapters 1, 9 and 10
Welfare assessment tools	Welfare assessment can encourage owner behaviour change if owners or the community are involved. They can be used to evaluate the impact on animals of other interventions, compared to an existing baseline	Owner buy-in to changes to their practices can be low if an auditor does the assessment with little owner involvement. Standardization requires on-going training and refreshers of welfare assessors to ensure reliability of results	Chapter 10, Case Study 1
Mentoring professionals	Mentoring is a more sustainable approach than providing free healthcare clinics. It can lead to systemic changes if used alongside changes to the education system	The reach is limited to individuals and depends on local capacity or international resources to fund and provide the mentors	Chapter 11

Undercover investigations	Investigation exposures can have high-impact media coverage and lead to public outcry, potentially resulting in closure or legally enforced changes for the locations involved or new legislation	These can be illegal depending on their nature and don't allow dialogue or influence. Their impact depends on the public response. Businesses won't want to respond to negative pressure unless it threatens their existence	Case Studies 2 and Behaviour change box
Owner consultation, group training class or workshops	Both knowledge and practice with demonstration can be covered. A high quality of welfare can be strived for owing to the level of individual attention. Small group sizes allow for an optimal coaching environment and dialogue between the owners	The reach is limited to the number of owners and animals an individual can work with. Owner compliance depends on the communication skills of the professional. Animals and owners may be unable to learn as they find a group environment too distracting	Chapters 2 and 4
Social marketing: print, TV or online media, websites, social media, podcasts	Large audiences can be reached to raise awareness of issues. Long-term changes can be achieved with repeated coverage leading to legislation or consumer purchasing changes	Awareness can be short-lived in societies with rapidly changing news and short attention spans in the digital age	Chapter 2

and to the case study contributors. Thank you to the animal welfare practitioners making the world a better place for animals, who were the inspiration for this book.

References

Appleby, M.C., Olsson, A.S. and Galindo, F. (eds) (2018) *Animal Welfare*, 3rd edn. CAB International, Wallingford, UK.

Balcombe, J.P., Barnard, N.D. and Sandusky, C. (2004) Laboratory routines cause animal stress. *Contemporary Topics in Laboratory Animal Science* 43(6), 42–51.

Bar-On, Y.M., Phillips, R. and Milo, R. (2018) 'The biomass distribution on Earth'. *Proceedings of the National Academy of Sciences* 115(25), 6506–6511. doi:10.1073/PNAS.1711842115

Boissy, A., Manteuffel, G., Jensen, M.B., Moe, R.O., Spruijt, B., Keeling, L.J. et al. (2007) Assessment of positive emotions in animals to improve their welfare. *Physiology and Behavior* 92, 375–397. doi:10.1016/j.physbeh.2007.02.003

Brambell, F.W.R. (1965) Report of the Technical Committee to Enquire Into the Welfare of Animals Kept Under Intensive Livestock Husbandry Systems, Fisheries (Bethesda). Her Majesty's Stationery Office, London.

Brudzynski, S.M. and Ociepa, D. (1992) Ultrasonic vocalization of laboratory rats in response to handling and touch. *Physiology and Behavior* 62(4), 655–660. doi:10.1016/0031-9384(92)90393-G

Clegg, I.L.K., Borger-Turner, J.L. and Eskelinen, H.C. (2015) C-Well: The development of a welfare assessment index for captive bottlenose dolphins (*Tursiops truncatus*). *Animal Welfare* 24, 267–282. doi:10.7120/09627286.24.3.267

Duncan, I.J. (1996) Animal welfare defined in terms of feelings. *Acta Agriculture Scandinavica Section A Animal Science* 27, 29–35.

AHAW, Nielsen, S.S. and Sihvonen, L.H. (2020) Scientific opinion concerning the killing of rabbits for purposes other than slaughter. *EFSA Journal* 18(1), 5943.

European Council (2017) Overview Report: Commercial Rabbit Farming in the European Union. Available at: https://ec.europa.eu/food/audits-analysis/overview_reports/act_getPDF.cfm?PDF_ID=1193 (accessed 30 March 2021).

Fraser, A.F. and Broom, D.M. (1990) *Farm Animal Behaviour and Welfare*. 3rd edition. CAB International, Wallingford, UK.

García Pinillos, R. (2018) *One Welfare: A Framework to Improve Animal Welfare and Human Wellbeing*. CAB International, Wallingford, UK.

Gärtner, K., Büttner, D., Döhler, K., Friedel, R., Lindena, J. and Trautschold, I. (1980) Stress response of rats to handling and experimental procedures. *Laboratory Animals*. doi:10.1258/002367780780937454

Grandin, T. (ed.) (2015) *Improving Animal Welfare: A Practical Approach*, 2nd edn. CAB International, Wallingford, UK.

LaFollette, M.R., O'Haire, M.E., Cloutier, S., Blankenberger, W.B. and Gaskill, B.N. (2017) Rat tickling: A systematic review of applications, outcomes, and moderators. *PLoS ONE* 12(4), e0175320. doi:10.1371/journal.pone.0175320

LaFollette, M.R., O'Haire, M.E., Cloutier, S. and Gaskill, B.N. (2018) Practical rat tickling: Determining an efficient and effective dosage of heterospecific play. *Applied Animal Behaviour Science* 208, 82–91. doi:10.1016/j.applanim.2018.08.005

LaFollette, M.R., Cloutier, S., Brady, C., Gaskill, B.N. and O'Haire, M.E. (2019) Laboratory animal welfare and human attitudes: A cross-sectional survey on heterospecific play or 'rat tickling'. *PLoS ONE* 14(8), e0220580. doi:10.1371/journal.pone.0220580

LaFollette, M.R., Cloutier, S., Brady, C.M., O'Haire, M.E. and Gaskill, B.N. (2020) Changing human behavior to improve animal welfare: A longitudinal investigation of training laboratory animal personnel about heterospecific play or 'rat tickling'. *Animals* 10(8), 1435.

Levitt, T. (2020) KFC admits a third of its chickens suffer painful inflammation. *The Guardian*, 30 July.

McMillan, F.D. (ed.) (2020) *Mental Health and Well-being in Animals, 2nd edn*. CAB International, Wallingford, UK.

Mellor, D.J. (2016) Moving beyond the 'five freedoms' by updating the 'five provisions' and introducing aligned 'animal welfare aims'. *Animals* 6(10), 59. doi:10.3390/ani6100059

Mellor, D.J. and Beausoleil, N.J. (2020) Moving beyond a problem-based focus on poor animal welfare toward creating opportunities to have positive welfare experiences. In: McMillan, F.D. (ed.) *Mental Health and Well-being in Animals*, 2nd edn. CAB International, Wallingford, UK, pp. 50–66.

Mellor, D.J., Beausoleil, N.J., Littlewood, K.E., McLean, A.N., McGreevy, P.D., Jones, B. and Wilkins, C. (2020) The 2020 Five Domains Model: Including human-animal interactions in assessments of animal welfare. *Animals* 10(10), 1870. https://doi.org/10.3390/ani10101870

Morgan, K.N. and Tromborg, C.T. (2007) Sources of stress in captivity. *Applied Animal Behaviour Science* 102, 262–302. doi:10.1016/j.applanim.2006.05.032

Rollin, B. (1992) *Animal Rights and Human Morality*. Prometheus Books, Buffalo, New York.

Sommerville, R., Ruiz, R. and Averós, X. (2017) A meta-analysis on the effects of the housing environment on the behaviour, mortality, and performance of growing rabbits. *Animal Welfare* 26(2), 223–238. doi:10.7120/09627286.26.2.223

Van der Stede, Y. and Winckler, C. (2020) Scientific Opinion on the health and welfare of rabbits farmed in different production systems. *EFSA Journal* 18(1), 5944. https://doi.org/10.2903/j.efsa.2020.5944

YouGov Plc (2020) 88% of UK public think cages are cruel. Available at: https://www.ciwf.org.uk/news/2020/12/88-of-uk-public-think-cages-are-cruel (accessed 30 March 2021).

Animal Welfare: The Human Element

2

Suzanne Rogers and Jo White
Human Behaviour Change for Animals CIC, UK

> If we do not understand why humans do the things they do, and what drives them to change, our potential to improve the lives of animals will not be met.

Human behaviour, what humans do, or don't do, is the root cause of most animal welfare problems. Therefore, to improve the lives of animals, it is important to understand behaviours in terms of the factors that cause them and maintain them, so that interventions can be designed that address the causes rather than the symptoms. The science of human behaviour change (HBC) can be applied not only to help us understand behaviour but also to change it. This chapter explores the different elements of HBC and illustrates why there is an increasing emphasis in the animal welfare field on learning about human, as well as other animal, behaviour.

Let's first consider our own experiences of behaviour change: please note down your answers to the following questions:

- Have you ever tried to change your behaviour? (e.g. Most of us at some time have wanted to eat less, exercise more or stop smoking)
- Did you have the knowledge needed to make the change? (e.g. Did you know what to eat, or how to exercise?)
- Did you have the motivation to change? (e.g. Did you understand the benefits of making the change? Most of us know that if we maintain a healthy weight, we might avoid certain health issues)
- Have you made and sustained the change? If so, was it easy? If not, then why do you think you did not manage to sustain the change?

A common misconception about how people process information is that raising awareness and providing information leads to behaviour change. Consider nutrition campaigns – it was considered that the majority of the population in the UK knows that it is recommended to eat five portions of fruit and vegetables a day, but in 2018 a UK government health survey showed that only 28% of people actually do eat that many portions (NHS Digital Services, 2020). Just because we know something, it does not mean we are going to change our behaviour and this is worth exploring because a stated aim of many projects is to increase awareness and knowledge of an issue with the assertion that this will lead to behaviour change. Another misconception is that changes in *attitude* will lead to behaviour change – in fact, it is entirely possible for people not to behave congruently with their attitudes. Attitudinal change can be important in the process of change but should not be used as an indicator for behaviour change. Furthermore, although intentions are considered a good predictor of behaviour, it is also common that people do not behave according to their *intentions*, something that we all have experience of ourselves!

As humans, we often understand the benefits of changing but despite having the relevant desire, knowledge, motivation and intentions, changing our behaviour is difficult. When it comes to our work to improve the lives of animals, however, we often assume that if we explain to people why they should change their behaviour to impact animal welfare positively, that they will instantly change accordingly and maintain that change. Consider, for example, a vet who explains to a client that their dog is obese and needs to lose weight to be healthy and avoid further exacerbating a health issue. This type of conversation does not always result in the animal being an ideal weight the next time they are brought into the surgery. The reasons why are complex and multifactorial, but even a basic understanding of human behaviour can help to increase compliance in such situations. It is clear, that given that the root cause of much animal suffering is human behaviour, we must better understand humans to effect change for animals.

To understand human behaviour we can consider many different fields of expertise (as illustrated in Fig. 2.1). The output of this huge body of work can

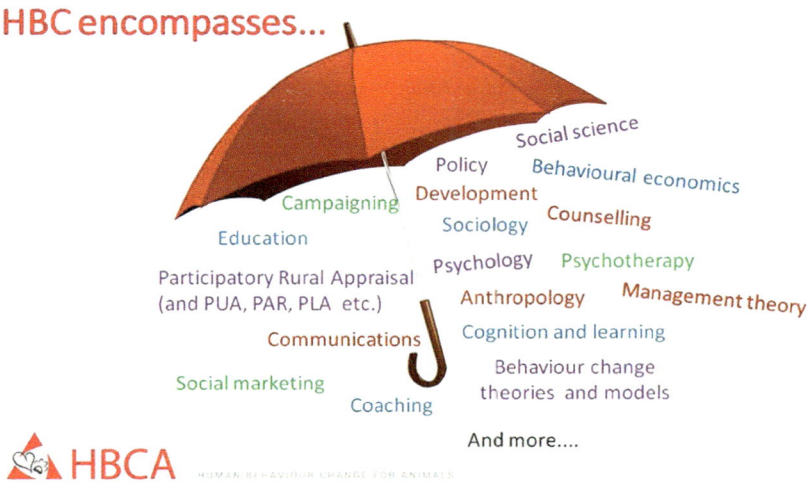

Fig. 2.1. Just some of the fields of research that include insights into human behaviour and how it might be influenced. (© Human Behaviour Change for Animals, 2020.)

be roughly summarized into four key principles (first described in White and Rogers, 2017): change is a process; understanding psychology is key in driving change; the environment influences change; and change must be owned. The principles overlap and various concepts fit across the principles – they provide a framework through which to consider the breadth and depth of the topic.

2.1 Principle 1: Change Is a Process

What causes people to change their behaviour, and what processes and stages are involved in behaviour change have been studied from many different angles and there are multitudes of models and frameworks that consider different aspects of this topic. There are various models that help to explain the behaviour that is, or isn't, taking place and then provide insight into how to change it. For example, the Transtheoretical Model (also known as the stages of change model) (Prochaska and DiClemente, 1984), suggests that change consists of five stages: pre-contemplation (where there is no awareness of the need to change), contemplation (when the need for change is being considered), preparation (in which measures are taken to prepare for change), action (changes are made) and maintenance (changes are maintained). This is not a linear process and behaviour can relapse at any point. Continuing with the example of how a veterinary surgeon might encourage change regarding an owner with an obese dog, if the owner is at the pre-contemplation stage, then they might need to be engaged by being asked what they know about the ideal weight of their breed of dog, and then provided with information about their animals' weight; this might result in a change of perception about what a healthy animal looks like. In this scenario, if the veterinarian were to focus on providing suggestions for actions the owner could take, they are unlikely to be successful because the owner is not at the stage to consider actions yet. Likewise, if the veterinarian were to focus on providing information about the need for the pet to lose weight when the owner already knows this and needs solutions, there is unlikely to be good compliance either. It is important not to offer various solutions that address assumed barriers but to determine the real barrier and address it accordingly.

The key message is that change is a process and we need to understand where people are in the process to be able to support them towards sustained change. Understanding what processes and triggers are relevant might help to move someone through the stages. For example, a veterinary practice aiming to apply the model to increase the number of clients that vaccinate their pets might create a strategy to move their clients through the stages: starting with pre-contemplation (e.g. clients receive a reminder for a booster vaccination in the post and put it somewhere safe); to contemplating doing something (e.g. clients actively plan to book an appointment or read the information about the need for vaccinations); through to preparation (booking an appointment); action (attending the appointment); and maintenance (vaccinating the following year). Taking these points into account might, for example, change the way veterinary practices market various prophylactic medicines, change the wording on the vaccination reminder, modify the appointment booking process and so on.

This model can also be applied at a community or societal level. For example, in terms of considering a strategic approach to introducing legislative change to ensure compliance, the model can be used to consider which stage the majority of the population are in – if it is in the contemplation stage or beyond, the public has an awareness of the issues and what to do to address them, and the introduction of legislation is more likely to be successful than if the majority of the population are in the pre-contemplation stage, and therefore are not even cognisant of any need for change. In that scenario, if legislation were introduced then it would be unlikely to be complied with. It could also be used as a tool for understanding and segmenting different parts of the population to ensure that they are communicated with in the right way; those who are pre-contemplation will not respond to the same messaging as those in other stages of change.

The stages of change model is useful and intuitive to use; for those who haven't considered behaviour change as a process before, it can be immensely helpful in providing a new framework upon which to map audiences or the development of understanding of an issue. At Human Behaviour Change for Animals, when the team needs to achieve a good understanding of a behaviour and how it could be changed, they sometimes use the COM-B model and Behaviour Change Wheel tool (Michie *et al.*, 2014). The COM-B model helps the team to understand a specific behaviour as being a result of the capability of the person to make the change (e.g. skills, knowledge), opportunity to make the change (e.g. social, environment) and motivational factors to make the change (e.g. automatic and reflective motivational factors). Once the team understands the behaviour they want to change, the Behaviour Change Wheel then builds on the understanding from the COM-B model to consider possible interventions and later policy elements too. The authors will not go into more detail in this chapter as Chapter 4 by Melissa Liszewski covers this tool in relation to an example for working equids.

Models that consider the relationship between emotion and behaviour, or between attitude, intention and behaviour are also important to consider.

2.2 Principle 2: Understanding Psychology Is Key in Driving Change

This principle explores areas such as how much change is someone's autonomous decision and how much is as a result of influence by others; how the mind works in learning and processing new information; what factors affect our motivation for change; how barriers for change are often very deep-seated beliefs and values, and how best to address this, and much more. Psychology is a huge topic, much of which is relevant to behaviour change. The authors will cover just four concepts here: confirmation bias, reactance, motivation and social norms.

2.2.1 Confirmation bias

We are more likely to take on information that fits with what we already know and our beliefs than information that challenges us – this is known in psychology as confirmation bias. If we enjoy visiting marine parks and believe that those who care for cetaceans in captivity meet all their needs, we are more likely to take on information that backs up this view than to take on information about animals struggling in confinement, for example. To avoid triggering this bias, we can focus on common or shared values: if we create dialogue focused on the similarities between ourselves and our audience by focusing on the values we share (e.g. the love of oceans and watching dolphins jump out of the water), we will have a foundation for more in-depth exploration of our differences.

2.2.2 Reactance

It is human nature, when faced with someone with a problem, to want to suggest possible solutions and to provide suggestions for ways to address the issue. In Motivational Interviewing (MI) (Miller and Rollnick, 2013), this human desire to provide solutions is known as the 'righting reflex'. However, when we make suggestions and provide ideas, counterintuitively it is likely to have the opposite of the intended effect. When faced with one side of an argument we are likely to bring up the other side, so you might generate more ideas against your solutions than you do support for them. This concept is termed 'reactance'. Also, by giving the client an opportunity to practise vocalizing reasons why not to change, for example, you enable those ideas to become more strongly held, or more embedded. Providing solutions also creates a dependency on the practitioner to keep providing solutions rather than the focus being on the client to suggest changes, or for suggestions to be co-created between client and practitioner. Providing solutions can, therefore, disempower your audience when you are aiming for the opposite result. Instead of providing solutions, we must develop skills that pave the way for members of our audience to come up with their own solutions and ideas, where we are the facilitators.

2.2.3 Motivation

If we have a better understanding of what motivates and influences people, we can apply the knowledge directly to our work. There are different 'camps' in this field, each with different perspectives about the primary drivers and how they interact, but it is useful to understand each view in the search for the best match for your work. Understanding the barriers to why some owners are reluctant to neuter their pets, for example, can provide ideas for how to remove those barriers. Another example might be to understand why someone is motivated to ride or compete on a horse even though the horse is lame or shows signs of pain. The reasons we might presume people would be motivated to do or not do something are very often not the same as the reasons they state, which are in turn often not the same as what is really going on.

Understanding the motivation for change and how new behaviours are abandoned or maintained is necessary in planning effective projects. An understanding of the relationship between behaviour change of individuals, and how that translates to increasing the dissemination of information and change throughout a community is vital in planning and adapting projects that rely on the spread of best practices.

2.2.4 Social norms

There are unwritten rules, informal understandings, that we all abide by regarding many aspects of our behaviour; these are known as social norms. For example, the distance it is considered 'acceptable' to stand from someone in a queue is a social norm that differs between cultures. Such behaviours can promote positive behaviours; for example, it is generally considered important to exercise your dog every day (in the UK). Social norms can also act as barriers to positive behaviours and promote the maintenance of negative behaviours. For example, keeping single rabbits in small hutches was a social norm in the UK for decades and has only recently been challenged by strong campaigns to better meet rabbits' needs. To encourage behaviours that are seen as going against the social norm can be challenging and requires a strategic approach. One element of this is to use a values-based approach, highlighting the similarities between people's values and using this to reframe the desired behaviour that is diverging from the norm. For example, when communicating about the sort of living space provisions rabbits need, a values-based focus first highlights the reason people keep rabbits and the shared joy of watching them perform certain behaviours. It then introduces the idea that if they are kept in a larger space than a typical hutch, those behaviours will be more easily observed as well as being better for the much-loved pet (Fig. 2.2).

2.3 Principle 3: The Environment Influences Behaviour

Our behaviour is influenced by environmental factors almost constantly. For example, simply introducing 'targets' in urinals was found to significantly

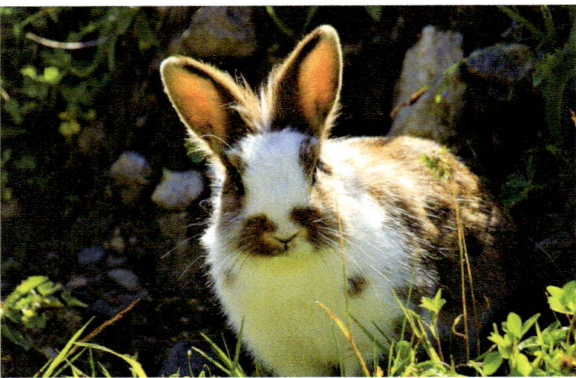

Fig. 2.2. The way that people keep rabbits is now moving away from keeping them singly in small hutches. (Photo by 'Lucas' copyright free from Pexels.)

improve sanitary conditions in public toilets, and during the COVID-19 pandemic environmental signals such as stickers on the ground significantly changed our queuing behaviours. Sometimes we do not have to engage directly with our audience to drive behaviour change – we can instead make changes to the environment that encourage the behaviour we want. An example where desired behaviour is encouraged through use of the environment is when the pet weigh bridge is placed in the waiting room at veterinary surgeries to encourage its use. An animal welfare example would be changing the choice of consumer products available (in the shopping environment) so that unhealthy products such as dog treats are less prominent and therefore less likely to be chosen over healthier alternatives. Another example is the introduction of innovative ways to dispose of rubbish on beaches, thus avoiding plastic pollution in the ocean – where artistic interactive sculptures that encourage responsible disposal of plastic bottles have been installed the number of bottles on the beaches has reduced (anecdotal reports).

As well as factors relating to the physical environment as described above, the policy environment also influences behaviour. The policy choices that are made and how they are enacted influences and affects behaviour. People can be coerced and restricted or incentivized through policy and legislative change. For example, restrictions influence people's behaviour regarding tail docking of dogs, whereas incentives influence people's behaviour regarding animal welfare labelling of farmed animal products.

2.4   Principle 4: Change Must Be 'Owned'

There is a saying, 'Tell me and I forget, show me and I remember, involve me and I truly understand', which perfectly illustrates this principle of change.

People need to truly appreciate the relevance of the desired behaviour change to them for change to happen.

If we consider the evidence that there is more to learning than people just being told what to do (e.g. providing resources, traditional top-down educational outreach), or just being shown what to do through a demonstration (e.g. demonstration of a handling or training technique), and, instead, we truly involve them in the process of change, we can facilitate that change. This process involves enabling people and communities to explore issues and come up with solutions themselves rather than 'train them' to implement a preconceived solution. For example, different veterinary clients respond to different ways of being 'engaged', they need different approaches to 'own' the change – some people like to ensure they understand everything in detail about their pet's diagnosis and treatment, others like to feel 'looked after' and do not want to know the details, some like to have an active role in monitoring their pet, and some would rather bring him/her to the vets more often. Assessing the client's personality to be able to involve them in the way that best fits their needs is an art and a science.

The field of MI applies this principle and is increasingly being used in the animal welfare sector to drive change. MI provides an evidence-based framework upon which to structure conversations about change. MI practitioners engage their clients in conversations using empathetic approaches. This enables the client to focus in on what they want and how to get there in an empowering way, which means the changes pledged are relevant to the client, specific for their situation and built towards making changes the clients are motivated to implement. Ultimately, the changes are 'owned'.

2.5 Change as a System

We are all part of a system of many interrelated parts, whether we are talking about our own bodies and how these different systems work together to make us function (e.g. the circulatory system, digestive system and so on), or the world we live in, as our actions, our behaviours, impact on each other and the world around us (e.g. the environment, the economy, spread of disease). So, to truly understand behaviour change, we must appreciate that behaviour operates in an interrelated system; we must consider everything as a whole, not in isolation. The causes of behaviour are multifactorial and are influenced by social factors such as culture, as well as the environmental context. It can be tempting to find one tool or framework that resonates with us in relation to a particular issue, and to want to apply a reductionist approach – considering behaviour change to be just about that single model and one process. However, no flow-chart style approach to behaviour change will work across all issues – we need to truly understand the behaviour we want to change before considering interventions. HBC research, therefore, seeks to fully understand an issue before selecting some of the many evidence-based frameworks and models through which to analyse the results and then structure an approach to designing interventions.

> Understanding human behaviour change is key to impactful interventions as people are the solution not just the problem. (HBCA)

2.6 The Role of Habits in Behaviour Change

Habits form a large part of our lives with around 40–45% of our daily behaviours being automatic habitual behaviour (e.g. looking at a mobile phone or cleaning our teeth in our morning routine) (Wood *et al.*, 2002). Many of the routine behaviours related to human–animal interaction, such as management and care, include habitual behaviours as the actions are repeated in the same context either automatically or with low levels of conscious thought (White, 2018). For example, once established, providing a specific type of enrichment during an animal's routine daily care, is an example of habitual behaviour because it is routinely performed, linked to the same contextual cues and requires limited active conscious effort to perform it. Human habits also affect animals in other ways; for example, our regular shopping behaviour is largely habitual and what we buy affects animals, whether directly in the case of animal products, or indirectly in the case of packaging that might end up polluting the environment.

In social marketing, there is a term 'behavioural prompts' that describes how new behaviours can be linked to parts of our established routine (our habits) to increase the chance of the behaviour being performed and becoming habitual. For example, physiotherapists have found clients to be much more likely to do the recommended exercises if they 'hook' them into their daily routine, and therefore most physiotherapists suggest that leg exercises are done when sitting on the toilet (the 'prompt') or making a cup of tea. This is supported by research that looks at the requirement to have a stable contextual cue for the habit to be formed (Lally *et al.*, 2010; Gardner, 2012; Stawarz *et al.*, 2014).

2.7 From Principles to Practice

Any project can be planned, researched, implemented and monitored in a way that applies the principles of HBC throughout all stages, through some parts or not at all. Figure 2.3 shows that a process that embraces HBC at all stages involves first understanding the issue (which includes testing assumptions, for example), then the intervention stage (change) and then the impact is assessed. Throughout all stages progress and activities are monitored and a research and development cycle approach is used, so that information gathered is used to tweak the project as it continues.

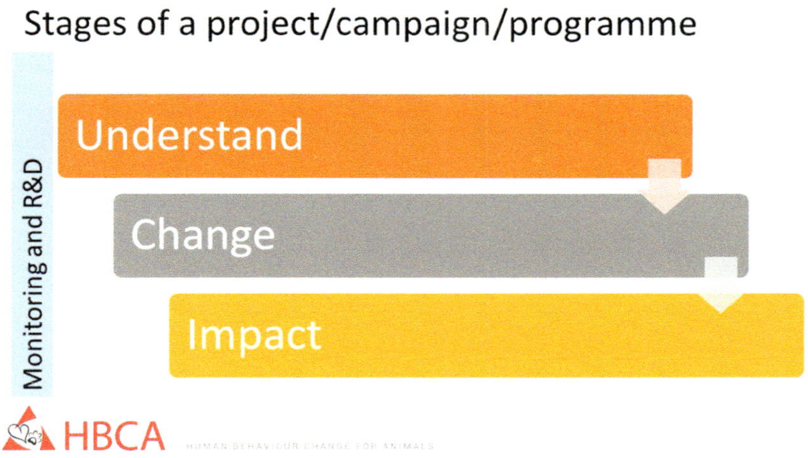

Stages of a project/campaign/programme

Monitoring and R&D
- Understand
- Change
- Impact

HBCA — HUMAN BEHAVIOUR CHANGE FOR ANIMALS

Fig. 2.3. The project process. (© Human Behaviour Change for Animals, 2020.)

Using an HBC-minded approach helps to mitigate the risk of negative unforeseen consequences. For example, several projects working towards ending the use of bears for entertainment in India and Pakistan focused on seizing the bears or persuading the owners to relinquish them, and then euthanizing the bears or moving them to a sanctuary as appropriate for each case. However, in some cases the owners would then get another bear, or a monkey or a snake to use for their street entertainment livelihood; the problem had not been addressed in a sustainable way and the welfare issue had 'moved to' another animal. In some cases, the owner had been supported to start a new livelihood such as a craft-making or recycling enterprise, but this new livelihood was not sustainable for some owners who enjoyed the entertainment aspect of the dancing bear livelihood and ultimately they would seek a way to go back into that work. More successful projects, however, considered the issue in a much more comprehensive way and recognized that the bear owners needed to be enthusiastic about any new proposed livelihood, and involved them in the process of choosing and setting up a new animal welfare-friendly business. It is vital to address a problem in a way that does not transfer welfare issues from one animal or species to another. See Chapter 10 for a case study.

An HBC-minded approach can be used in all parts of the project from the way stakeholders are identified and engaged, to the communication ethos used, to empowering people involved, and much more. Activities are not HBC or an alternative approach, but can incorporate HBC thinking; for example, educational materials could be produced in an HBC-minded way by consideration of what pictures are used, how they are sourced, how the content is sourced, how the material can include interactive elements and how they involve the person.

2.8 Summary

HBC is a huge topic and it is impossible to comprehensively introduce all the relevant concepts in one chapter. The key take-home messages are:

- To address the cause of animal welfare issues we must consider the human element.
- There is no single process or approach to change human behaviour; however, key principles can be considered that fit with the ethos and premise of the approach.
- We must avoid making assumptions about why people do, and don't do, behaviours that affect animals, and find out through research and engagement. Otherwise we will design interventions in a way that does not address the true causes of unwanted behaviour or break down the true barriers to performing the desired behaviours.
- The application of the science of HBC needs to be considered as a system with many different components.
- Using an HBC-minded approach helps to mitigate the risk of negative unforeseen consequences.
- HBC can be used throughout every stage of a project from conception, through planning, implementation and assessment, or to inform particular aspects of a piece of work.

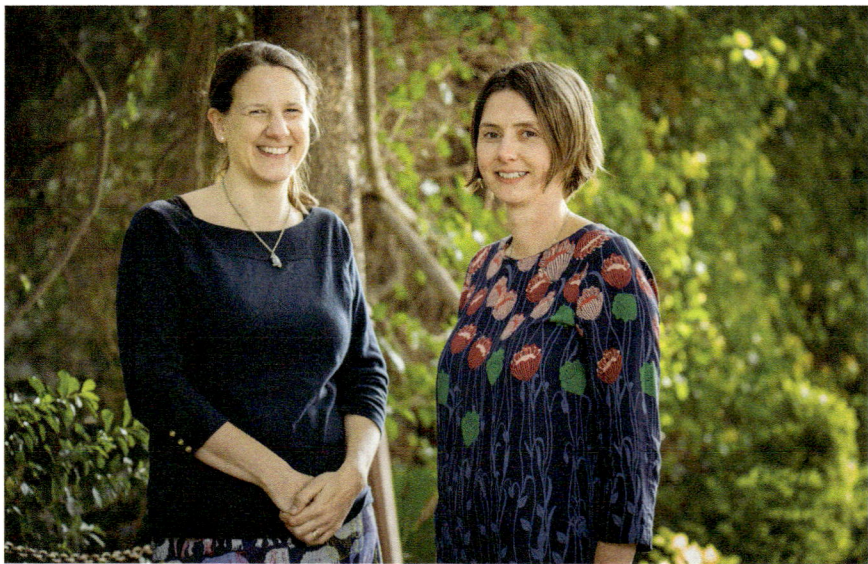

Fig. 2.4. The authors Suzanne and Jo (© Jo-Anne McArthur, Unbound.)

Case Study 1: Comprehensive Humane Dog Population Management Programmes, the Human Element

In many countries roaming dogs are a ubiquitous part of communities and, in some places, live in harmony with humans. However, problems are also common where humans and street dogs share an environment. There is a huge range of factors to consider when attempting to understand the complexities of issues that arise in communities with roaming dogs, and these factors can affect both dog and human welfare. For example, there are public health concerns (e.g. regarding dog waste and disease transmission), ecological factors (e.g. dogs posing a risk to native wildlife), political, cultural and religious attitudes (e.g. differing attitudes towards euthanasia of very sick dogs), issues with behaviour of dogs to humans (e.g. chasing or barking), issues regarding the behaviour of humans towards dogs (e.g. pouring hot water on dogs who approach their property) and issues affecting dog health (e.g. lack of appropriate food, skin disease).

The use of sterilization for controlling stray animal populations was first suggested and implemented in the 1960s. In the following decades, neutering became an increasing used tool to try to address some of the issues with roaming dogs – mostly the assumption that there are 'too many' and that decreasing the numbers would solve the issues. Immense passion and considerable resources went into funding and implementing neutering programmes, but it gradually became apparent that programmes focused on neutering alone sometimes created problems in themselves. In some cases, animals who were much-loved pets allowed to roam were 'kidnapped' for neutering against the wishes or without the knowledge of the owners, and not returned to where they came from. There were also concerns that removing dogs from one area merely enabled other dogs to 'move in' to that area and that enabling puppies to live for longer by supporting their health ultimately increased the population. In some cases, appropriate post-operative care was causing very visible welfare issues and, without the support of the communities, programmes were often treated with suspicion.

In 2006, six of the leading animal welfare organizations came together as the International Companion Animal Management (ICAM) coalition in recognition of the need for dog population management programmes to become more strategic. They produced guidelines for each stage of a programme from the methodology for measuring dog population sizes and assessing if any intervention was needed (sometimes the perception from outsiders that there are 'too many dogs' is not seen as a problem by the community, for example), to how to engage various stakeholders, to best working practices of running interventions, to how to monitor and evaluate the impact of programmes. They created a community through which projects could share their experience and ideas as well as seek support and help implementing the guidelines. Crucially, the group recognized the importance of understanding the human element of roaming dog issues. Their surveys and questionnaires were innovative in how they sought to truly understand the attitudes and behaviours towards roaming dogs in each individual context. They appreciated that if you make assumptions about what people's attitudes are, or why they behave in a certain way, and get them wrong then you will be working to address barriers that don't reflect the real barriers and waste your resources. They recognized the importance of involving local stakeholders – the importance of working with the authorities towards a common aim of addressing key issues; working with local vets rather than undercutting them using project vets; working with the community (no more dog-napping!), and so on. By understanding the importance of human behaviour as part of the problem they used it to be also part of the solution.

How to Change the Behaviour of Stakeholders: A Guide

Participatory exercise: the cobweb of needs (Fig. 2.5)

Participatory exercises can be undertaken with various stakeholders to explore an issue and possible solutions. This exercise has been used in many different contexts and cultures and is always popular. It enables the exploration of the current welfare state of individual animals, or a population of animals, and provides a breakdown of how better to meet the animals' needs.

For this example, we can consider the needs of a working equid.

1. Ask the group 'What does a horse need?' Pick one need at a time.
2. For the first need, draw a symbol (or ask a volunteer to draw a symbol) on a card to represent that need (e.g. a bucket of water). These cards are the blue cards in the photograph.

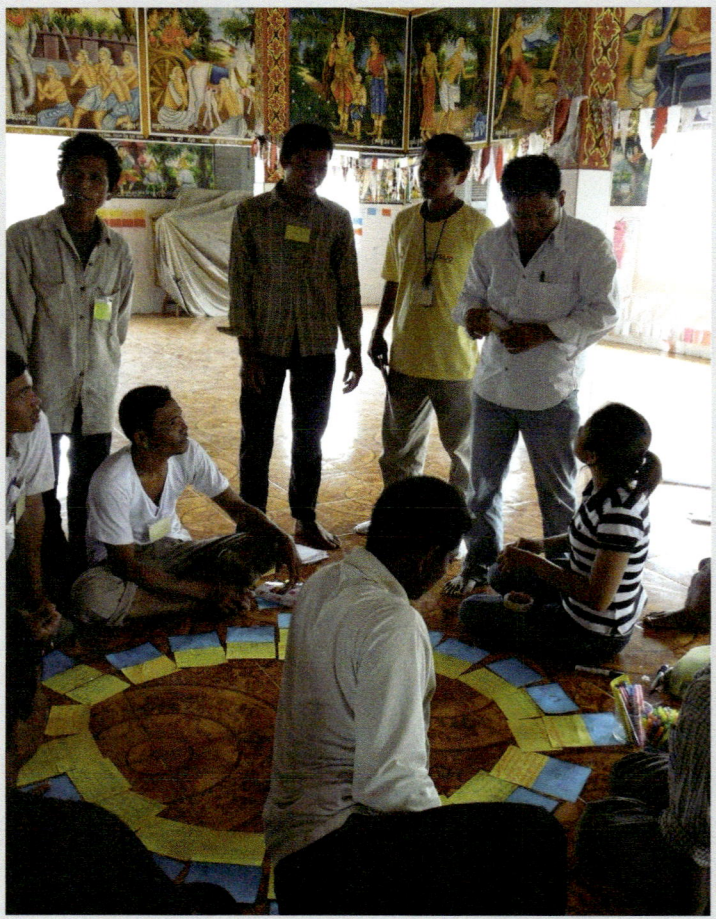

Fig. 2.5. The cobweb of needs. (© Human Behaviour Change for Animals, 2020.)

Continued

Continued.

3. Ask the group for details relating to that need (in an ideal situation, *not* the current situation) and on a second card (yellow cards in the photograph) write the list of criteria (e.g. clean water, clean bucket, offer water regularly). The more criteria the better because these can be used later to show how small changes can be made to improve things for the animal if bigger changes are too daunting.

4. Place both cards ('need' card and 'criteria' card) together as shown in the picture. Ask for a second need and repeat stages 1–4 until approximately 20 needs have been identified (to cover all aspects of management and work).

5. Lay out the pairs of cards in a circle and place a marker at the centre (see picture).

6. Identify the 'level' the need is met for a particular horse, or the 'average' horse in a community, by placing a marker between the centre of the circle and the card. The closer the marker is to the outside of the circle, the more common it is for the criteria to be met for the animal; if the marker is at the centre then none of the criteria for that need is often met.

7. Transfer the cards onto paper and join up the marker points to form the line of the 'spider's web' as shown in in Fig. 2.6.

8. Optional extra stage: Explore potential impacts of each 'need' on poor welfare. Score out of 10 using seeds or beans, where greater numbers of seeds indicate a greater potential for poor welfare. Place the piles of seeds around the edge of the circle.

9. Discuss changes that can be made to better meet the animal's needs. Note that the criteria on the second cards provide incremental changes to be made. Discuss and plan which changes to prioritize, when to reconvene to discuss changes

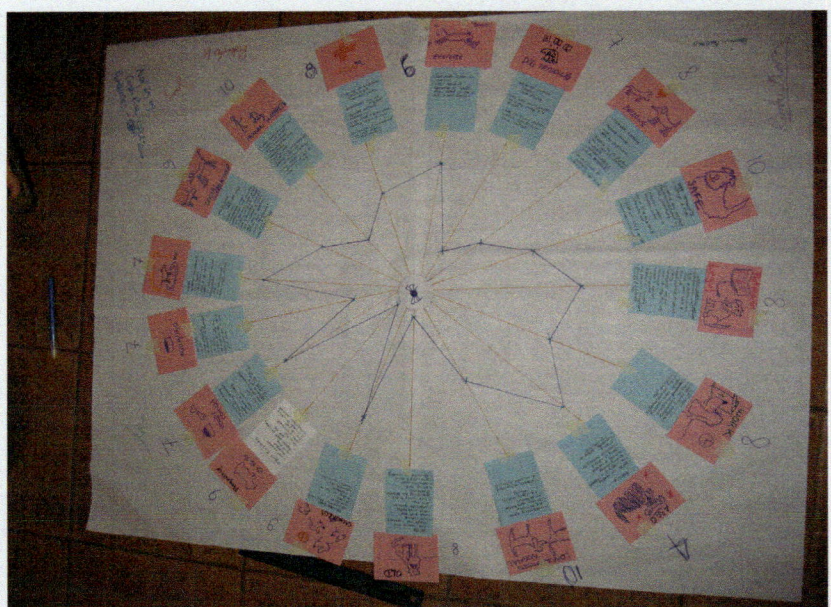

Fig. 2.6. The cobweb of needs: a personal development exercise. (© Human Behaviour Change for Animals, 2020.)

Continued

> Continued.
>
> made and so on. This stage will depend on the context and audience you are doing the exercise with.
>
> Note: an example of a context for this exercise was in a rabbit welfare workshop with rabbit owners in the UK. The Human Behaviour Change for Animals team first asked participants to place the markers for the average rabbit in the UK as a group then to repeat it for their own pet rabbit (individually). The group was then supported to enact the changes identified over the course of the project.
>
> This exercise could also be used as a personal development exercise with different areas of a person's life around the edge (e.g. technical knowledge, practical skill set, job satisfaction, human behaviour skills, interpersonal skills, outreach work, work–life balance and so on) or as an exercise to explore the needs of different parts of an organization.

References

Gardner, B. (2012) Habit as automaticity, not frequency. *The European Health Psychologist* 14(2), 32–36. doi:10.1037/e544772013-003

Lally, P., van Jaarsveld, C.H.M., Potts, H.W.W. and Wardle, J. (2010) How are habits formed: Modelling habit formation in the real world. *European Journal of Social Psychology* 40(6), 998–1009. https://doi.org/10.1002/ejsp.674

Michie, S., Atkins, L. and West, R. (2014) *The Behaviour Change Wheel: A Guide to Designing Interventions.* Silverback Publishing, London.

Miller, W.R. and Rollnick, S. (2013) *Motivational Interviewing: Helping People Change. Applications of Motivational Interviewing*, 3rd edn. Guilford Press, New York.

NHS Digital Services (2020) Health Survey for England 2018. Available at: https://digital.nhs.uk/data-and-information/publications/statistical/health-survey-for-england/2018/final-page-copy-2 (accessed 28 August 2020).

Prochaska, J.O. and DiClemente, C.C. (1984) *The Transtheoretical Approach: Towards a Systematic Eclectic Framework.* Dow Jones Irwin, Homewood, Illinois.

Stawarz, K., Cox, A.L. and Blandford, A. (2014) Beyond self-tracking and reminders: Designing smartphone apps that support habit formation. CHI 2015 Conference Paper. Seoul, Republic of Korea. doi:10.1145/2702123.2702230

White, J.S. (2018) Human behaviour change to improving animal welfare through habit formation. Unpublished Master's thesis, Derby University, Derby, UK.

White, J. and Rogers, S. (2017, September) Keynote Presentation: Making animal welfare sustainable – Human Behaviour Change for Animal Behaviour: The human element. In: Denenberg, S. (ed.) *Proceedings of the 11th International Veterinary Behaviour Meeting*, Samorin, Slovakia, September 2017. CAB International, Wallingford, UK, pp. 54–58.

Wood, W., Quinn, J.M. and Kashy, D.A. (2002) Habits in everyday life: thought, emotion, and action. *Journal of Personality and Social Psychology* 83(6), 1281–1297. doi:10.1037//0022-3514.83.6.1281

From Stakeholder Education to Engagement, Using Strategies from Social Science

3

Beth Ventura[1] and Erica Hogstad Fjæran[2]

[1]*Department of Animal Science, University of Minnesota, St. Paul, Minnesota, USA;* [2]*Foreningen Norske Etologer (Association of Norwegian Ethologists), Steinkjer, Norway*

3.1 Setting the Stage

Animal welfare affects and engages most people, and in the broadest sense is essential to individual lives, food production and environmental sustainability, among other considerations (Pinillos, 2018). Animal welfare is a multifaceted science, encompassing physiology, anatomy, nutrition, genetics, behaviour, cognition, medicine and human–animal interactions, among many other considerations. Such a spectrum offers occasional contradictions between fields of expertise, which often result in different ideas and ethical perspectives relative to how welfare should be defined and assessed. Given such context, even scientists and other educated practitioners are bound to differ in their opinions or priorities regarding animal welfare.

That a range of perspectives exists for what constitutes a good quality of life for an animal is underscored by the diverse interpretations of animal welfare in the literature (e.g. Broom, 1991; Duncan, 1993; Rollin, 1993). Fraser *et al.*'s (1997) theory of animal welfare as three distinct but interrelated aspects provides a useful framework to understand these values (Fig. 3.1). This framework suggests that welfare has to do with an animal's: *biological functioning* (how an animal physically functions), *affective state* (how an animal feels) and *natural living* (the degree to which an animal lives a natural life). Considering this, aiming for consensus on a 'correct' understanding of animal welfare may prove difficult. Yet by recognizing and naming such complexity and diversity in interpretations, stakeholders can more effectively communicate within and across diverse groups.

Those who work with animals (referred to here as 'practitioners' and who include but certainly are not limited to veterinarians, farmers, ethologists, animal scientists and professionals like trainers, zookeepers and welfare

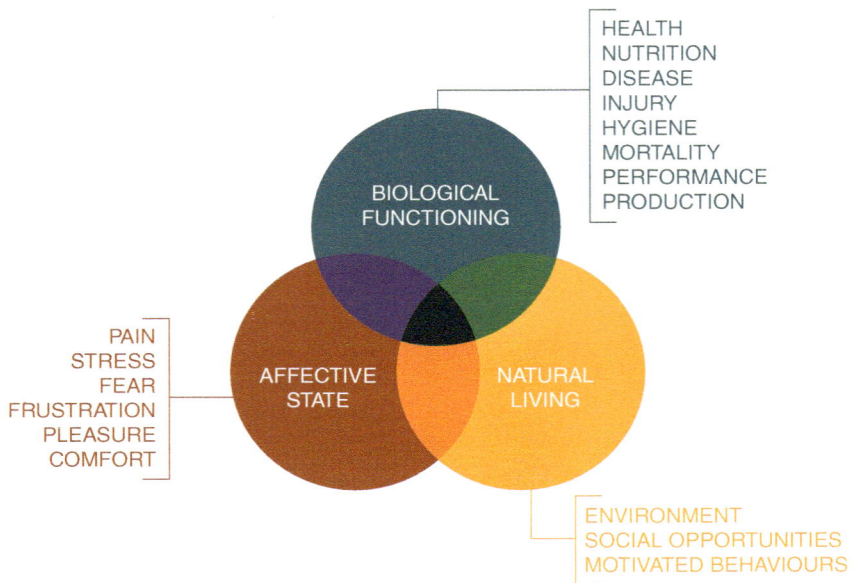

Fig. 3.1. Three spheres framework for animal welfare, Fraser et al. (1997). (Image: Turid Saursaunet.)

advocates) and members of the public who use animals (functioning as consumers, customers, owners, clients and citizens) often differ in their views relative to how those animals should be cared for and managed. Yet both practitioners and the public contribute to societal conversations and decisions affecting animals. Practitioners are often considered as experts in recognition of the unique set of knowledge and experience gained through their training and professional work. At the same time, the public also function as stakeholders in that they both impact and are impacted by animals, for example, through their guardianship of pets, consumption of animal products, expression of conservation behaviours, and voices in social and political processes that impact animals.

The nature of working in animal welfare necessitates that practitioners must frequently connect with members of the public. This relationship occurs in part as an effort to bridge the gap between identifying best management practices and ensuring implementation by targeting and changing the behaviour of people who directly use and impact animals. Often, this connection takes the form of knowledge translation from animal expert to lay person; for example, to address false assumptions about husbandry practices on farms or correct potentially harmful pet–owner interactions. While knowledge translation remains an important goal, this chapter will examine the challenges that arise when attempts to engage the public rest on one-way education alone. Rather, animal practitioners may benefit from a reimagining of what effective public engagement to improve animal welfare may look like.

3.2 Challenges to Effective Engagement

3.2.1 Public knowledge, awareness and information access

Despite being the focus of much conversation, there is relatively little research on the specifics of what the public knows and understands about animal welfare. What knowledge does exist suggests that public understanding of animal welfare is complicated and dependent on many factors (Evans and Miele, 2019).

With respect to farm animal welfare, most research suggests that knowledge, at least in practical terms, is relatively low. For example, the 2007 Eurobarometer survey identified that the majority of over 29,000 EU citizens surveyed across 25 member states claimed little to no knowledge of husbandry practices. A decade later, the 2016 Eurobarometer did not ask people to self-assess their knowledge but did identify that most expressed the desire to know more about how farmed animals are raised. Other work on specific industries likewise suggests that lay people report knowing little about livestock production (e.g. Ellis *et al.*, 2009; Cummins *et al.*, 2015; see Fig. 3.2).

A similar story appears with respect to what people know about other species. For example, a diverse panel of experts in the UK identified lack of owner knowledge about pet behaviour and health and failure to seek expert care as top animal welfare priorities (Rioja-Lang *et al.*, 2020). North American surveys have likewise found variable and often poor behavioural knowledge in cat

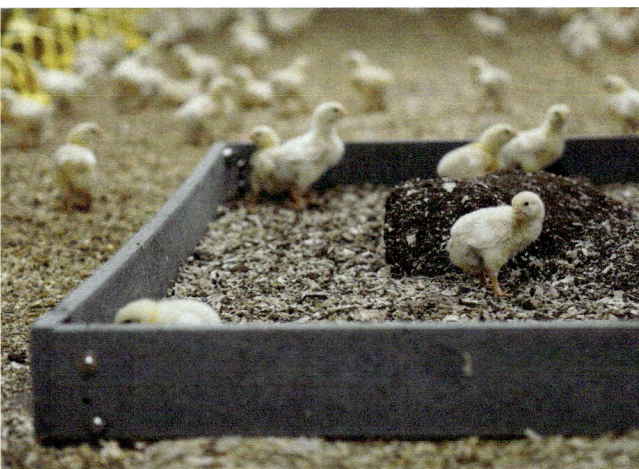

Fig. 3.2. Farming practices to promote natural behaviour in broiler rearing is mandatory in Norway. Environmental enrichment is an increasingly important measure to improve animal welfare. Measures brought on by research in the animal science field contribute to better lives of farm animals, but are not always well known to the public. (Photo: Erica Hogstad Fjæran.)

and dog owners, though those with advanced knowledge or training reported better detection of problem behaviours (Jacobs et al., 2017) and fewer behavioural problems in their pets (Grigg and Kogan, 2019).

Compounding this problem, there are some reports that much of the public lacks any source of animal welfare information and may be reluctant to access new knowledge, instead choosing to pursue wilful ignorance (McKendree et al., 2014; Bell et al., 2017). There are, however, some promising indications that animal welfare scientists are perceived as having trustworthy information and priorities (Evans and Miele, 2019).

Considering such reports of limited knowledge and pending more research about how much the public *actually knows*, poor public understanding may contribute to conflict between animal practitioners and the public.

3.2.2 Cognitive biases relative to animals

Another challenge is the reality that people are challenged by their own biases and preconceived notions of how animals live, learn and handle challenges. Confronting one's own perceptual barriers about animal welfare is a hurdle to overcome for anyone, even those well acquainted with animal welfare science.

Human minds are designed to simplify attempts at dealing with the world by applying rules of thumb to process information (*heuristics*). Such mental shortcuts reduce the effort of decision making and can be an efficient way of arriving at a conclusion. Yet heuristics can also be a kind of cognitive laziness. People can, for example, substitute simpler but related questions in place of more complex, difficult questions (*attribute substitution*). In terms of animal welfare knowledge, or lack thereof, such shortcuts may lead to false assumptions (e.g. by incorrectly transferring welfare indicators from one animal species to another). Likewise, people may be challenged by *anchoring biases*, or the tendency to rely too heavily on the first piece of information learned. This may then create false certainty in what someone thinks they know about animal welfare. Others may be challenged in their favouring of information that conforms to existing beliefs and discounting of evidence that does not. Such *confirmation biases* may limit one's knowledge foundation by hindering one from exploring or accepting alternative solutions (Kahneman, 2011).

The issue of addressing problem behaviour in dogs illuminates how these biases may play out to the detriment of animal welfare. Early studies of captive wolves were long the baseline for behavioural comparisons of dominance in the domestic dog, yet these have been more recently debunked by more careful observation of both dogs and wolves. Unfortunately, some trainers are still influenced by outdated theories, advising dog owners to 'take charge' as pack leaders and use aversive training methods that flood dogs with stressful situations. Such approaches generally include little focus on stress mitigation and can generate avoidance, fear, pain and/or aggression (Ziv, 2017). If these methods are someone's first introduction to dog training, however, they are likely to become their *anchoring bias*. Following this, *confirmation biases* will prompt inclinations to seek additional sources supporting outdated thinking. And as the mind favours simplifications (*heuristics*), the tendency to fall for shortcuts to achieve desired behaviour is likely to follow.

Adding to these biases is the tendency to compare human and animal traits. By *anthropomorphizing* animals, people may incorrectly interpret an animal's needs and behaviours in the disfavour of the animal's welfare (Serpell, 2019). For example, some owners perceive dog behaviour as 'guilty' in certain situations, believing that dogs know when they have committed a disapproved act (Hecht *et al.*, 2012). However, behavioural analysis has revealed no difference between obedient and disobedient dogs after having the opportunity to break a rule in owners' absences. Perhaps a better approach then is to apply anthropomorphistic theories with caution, recognizing that even though attributing human-like traits to non-human animals may sometimes be of partial value, it may just as well both over- and underestimate animals' abilities (Williams *et al.*, 2020).

3.2.3 Animal practitioners and experts

In addition to informational and cognitive biases in members of the public as well as in themselves, animal practitioners must also reckon with the following:

Science and 'facts' are the language of experts. Many animal practitioners, as with scientific experts, are trained to rely on science as the most effective and desirable basis from which to improve practice and make change (Simis *et al.*, 2016). The impulse of the expert may then be to assume that 'the science' should be the only language in which to communicate about issues requiring change. That experts' worldviews rest firmly on scientific foundations is essential and should not change. However, as much of the public has not received similar training, experts may find themselves operating on different wavelengths from the public. It is difficult to cross such a gap without the help of an additional language.

Experts will benefit from learning new languages. Science has long been embedded in social structures (Simis *et al.*, 2016). The field of animal welfare exemplifies this as a science born out of societal mandates to address the treatment of animals and that consequently has ethical, legal, political and social ramifications (Fraser *et al.*, 1997). The inherently interdisciplinary nature of animal welfare science, then, reflects a need for its practitioners to be versed in languages that will help them navigate this complexity. However, many in the veterinary and animal fields have traditionally lacked formal training in psychology, sociology and communication (McDermott *et al.*, 2017). Such training would ensure that practitioners better understand 'the processes by which citizens arrive at opinions and how to communicate effectively with such audiences' (Simis *et al.*, 2016, p. 403). Without such training, communication efforts may not work, especially if they rest on outdated assumptions about how people process information about animals.

Experts 'other' the public by assuming them ignorant of their language. It is common for those working with animals to ascribe ignorance on behalf of the public. For example, farmers and veterinarians have often described the public as ignorant and as having unrealistic, inappropriate expectations for animal care (Benard and de Cock Buning, 2013; Buddle *et al.*, 2021; Ventura *et al.*, in preparation). That experts assume the public is ignorant of the science and practices within one's field is nothing new, and animal practitioners are certainly not the only ones to do it. Such an assumption is common in discourse about public roles in science and is well described in the knowledge deficit model (Wynne and Irwin, 1996).

Assumption of the deficit model continues to frame how many experts approach public engagement about science-related matters (Simis *et al.*, 2016). A key part of the deficit model is the assumption that when experts make recommendations, defend practices or otherwise hinge communications based on science, if the public does not accept what they are told, it is because they do not understand the science and by extension the reality of the situation. The deficit model thus assumes that public concerns require correction. Often the approach has been to take up this gap through one-way education efforts designed to bring public opinion in line with expert views (Hansen *et al.*, 2003; Simis *et al.*, 2016).

3.3   Rectifying the Expert–Public Gap

The question then becomes: are animal experts' own beliefs about public ignorance fully justified? In many cases, the answer is likely 'yes'. Communication on matters related to animal care, behaviour and welfare must continue to share information grounded in science. However, animal practitioners stand to improve the value and impact of their communication efforts if they can re-evaluate this 'othering' of the public, as continuing to do so may limit or even prevent meaningful engagement (see Simis *et al.*, 2016). Assumptions about public ignorance are a poor foundation for animal welfare communication, for the following reasons:

- The deficit model fails to recognize that people evaluate issues and make decisions not just on the basis of information, but also as a result of their past lived experiences, their social and familial groups, and their cultural backgrounds. Importantly, people may disagree with or reject expert consensus because it does not align with their core values (see Hansen *et al.*, 2003). Thus, acknowledging that communication of science alone may fail to change minds may be a first step in establishing effective engagement around a value-laden topic such as animal welfare.
- It remains a possibility that forcing information that conflicts with people's underlying values may cause them to cling more firmly to their original beliefs (*the backfire effect*; Nyhan and Reifler, 2010). Though this phenomenon has been called into question (Wood and Porter, 2016), what remains clear is that people tend to seek ways to reduce cognitive burden, which may have unintended consequences if the goal is to 'educate the public' about animal issues. There is also some evidence that providing information about some animal topics (like farming) can provoke increased concern

(Ryan *et al.*, 2015; Ventura *et al.*, 2016, 2020). Perhaps not the backfire effect exactly, but certainly undesirable for anyone wishing to share their story about their approach to animal care.

> **Case Study 1: Animal Welfare Is Personal**
>
> Animal welfare is a multifaceted topic that brings about strong emotional responses. Many of these emotions originate in a primal part of the brain called the amygdala, which humans share with most other animals. The amygdala is essential to survival and prepares the body for behaviours such as fight, flight and freeze. Yet in humans our brain translates even the thought of stress (like engaging in an emotional topic such as animal welfare) into an activation of alert mode (Nordengen, 2019). In other words, taking in new knowledge and learning from others may be especially difficult when it relates to matters close to the heart, simply because one's own body physiologically and emotionally battles the new idea.
>
> The human behaviour of caring for others relates to the sociality of our species, and to critique such can easily provoke emotional responses. As pets today are often viewed as family members, appraisals on their treatment and training are likely to be regarded as direct offences to one's life and choices. Similarly, animals on a farm are part of a farmer's identity and life, to which questions and critique can be met with scepticism or even resentment.
>
> What may be well-intended advice may get lost in translation and perceived as presumptuous, assaulting or rejected altogether. Such emotional defensive responses are the result of animal welfare being an inherent part of human identity.

- Finally, 'the public' is not a single entity. People invariably have diverse views and reactions to receiving new information, a direct result of their varied backgrounds, cultures and values. So while information provision may bring some people into agreement with the communicator's objectives and values, the same content is likely to have an opposing effect on another segment of people. Accounting for different segments of the public and tailoring communications and expectations of outcomes accordingly is therefore recommended.

> **Case Study 2: Values and Reactions to Learning About Animal Welfare Are Diverse**
>
> Opportunities to observe segmentation in public attitudes to animal welfare are everywhere, and are especially well documented with respect to livestock (e.g. Vanhonacker *et al.*, 2007; Verbeke, 2009; Evans and Miele, 2019). It should come as no surprise then that diverse reactions also occur when lay people learn more about animal welfare. For example, though nearly all study participants ($n = 50$) who toured a university dairy farm in Canada learned more about the mechanics of dairy production, not everyone came away happier about dairy farming. Rather, just 24% improved their perceptions while 33% became more critical, a split in perception that was associated with whether the new information aligned or conflicted with existing values for animal welfare (Ventura *et al.*, 2016).
>
> Such segmentation of judgement after being exposed to the same set of information and conditions is likely to have profound consequences for any effort to influence

Continued

Case Study 2: Continued.

public behaviour about animal welfare, illustrated by another anecdote: as part of a learning module in a class about animals and society, undergraduate students ($n = 300$/class) at the University of Minnesota spend a week learning about laying hen husbandry and egg production. All students are exposed to the same information about system impacts on welfare, worker safety and sustainability; asked to complete an exercise to analyse US egg labels; and share how they plan to approach their egg-purchasing behaviour in future (Fig. 3.3). Year after year, students diverge in their decisions, underscoring how diversely individuals digest the same information.

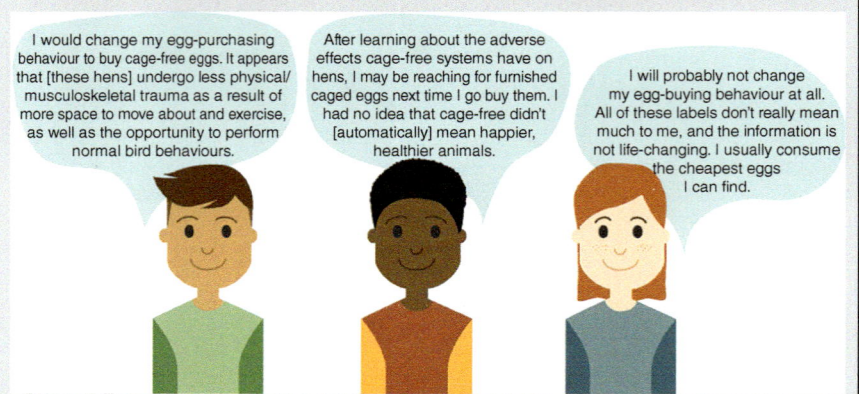

Fig. 3.3. American university students differ in their behavioural intentions to purchase eggs after learning the same information about the laying hen industry. (Image: Turid Saursaunet.)

3.4 Moving Forward

The desired outcome, then, is for increased alignment between experts and the public, which will inevitably mean compromises in both directions. To be sure, increased uptake of expert recommendations for animal welfare is crucial. Achieving this will require animal practitioners to more readily seek out where shared values exist between themselves and their target audience. Using Fraser *et al.*'s (1997) animal welfare framework, the public strongly privileges issues related to natural living as paramount to animal welfare, in contrast to the relatively lesser importance ascribed by many animal practitioners (e.g. veterinarians and farmers; Evans and Miele, 2019; Proudfoot and Ventura, 2020). However, practitioners are also cautioned to avoid falsely dichotomizing animal welfare values as 'expert vs public'. Indeed, many experts also prioritize natural living, while the public also values biological functioning and affective states and hence agrees with expert emphasis on the importance of these areas (see Ventura, 2015). Animal practitioners are thus encouraged to keep in mind that agreement between themselves and non-practitioners on many animal welfare topics may already exist (see Verbeke, 2009; Averós *et al.*, 2013).

In concluding this chapter, there are some tips in the following box on how practitioners can better bridge any remaining gaps between themselves and the public towards the improvement of animal welfare. These strategies are recommended as needed 'first steps' to take before one can hope to change stakeholder behaviour.

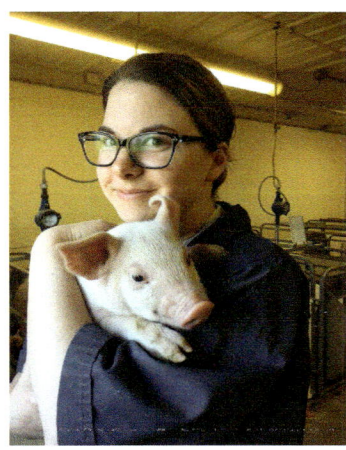
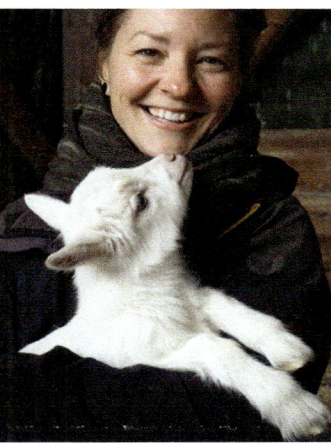

Fig. 3.4. Authors Beth and Erica.

How to Change the Behaviour of Public Stakeholders

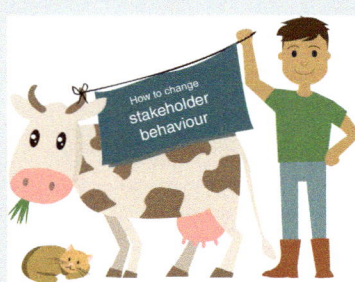

(Image: Turid Saursaunet.)

1. Develop knowledge of the social sciences, effective communication skills and complementary animal welfare sciences. As many animal practitioners often lack formal communication training (Mossop *et al.*, 2015, Simis *et al.*, 2016), individual practitioners are encouraged to pursue communication training and to read the literature on animal welfare attitudes, public acceptance of science and theories of behaviour change. Those in charge of curriculum planning likewise should implement coursework on these subjects as a core part of training future practitioners well placed to meet the demands of a field situated within competing and complicated societal perspectives. Furthermore, a robust animal welfare science should itself encourage a more interdisciplinary, collaborative approach for all practitioners. Ethologists in particular stand to serve as well-equipped scientists in the field of behaviour, both of human and non-human animals, thus serving in part as liaisons to change human behaviour to improve animal welfare.

2. Use strategic communication techniques to identify where shared values exist and practice adaptive transparency to seek alignment with those values.

Continued

Continued.

Practitioners are encouraged to practice *adaptive transparency*; that is, to information-share the hows and whys behind animal management recommendations and practices (the transparency part), and then be prepared to listen, respond and potentially modify practices based on how the public respond to receiving information.

Ask questions like 'What does good animal welfare look like to you?' and 'Can you share the reasons behind your belief in "X"?' Listening to the responses that emerge with the intent to understand, without interrupting or interjecting, and then summarizing back to the speaker is part of a practice of *reflective listening* (see Shaw, 2006). Practitioners are also encouraged to engage in *frame reflection* such that they place themselves in the position of the other person and interrogate how they would believe, think or feel in that position (Schön and Rein, 1994). Frame reflection has been shown to increase one's own capacity to learn within a different perspective about animals (Benard and de Cock Buning, 2013) and can improve practitioner belief in the legitimacy of other perspectives, setting the stage for more fruitful dialogues about animal welfare (Proudfoot and Ventura, 2020). Cultivating these practices will also help create non-judgemental spaces for open dialogue, where people feel empowered to share their perspectives without fear of seeming ridiculous. The construction of such spaces is key in building better relationships between animal practitioners and the public, and as a bonus, may make people more likely to listen and apply recommendations. Collectively, these practices will also enable better understanding of the values underlying someone's concerns, if and where any shared values exist, and where genuine knowledge gaps exist, thus helping the expert to target communications more specifically to influence decisions that impact welfare.

3. *Acknowledge compromises in animal welfare.* Practitioners may also benefit by acknowledging that the complexity of animal welfare implies that improving welfare in one respect may hinder efforts to improve it in another. Dogs, for example, are often kept home alone and walked on a leash because of work and safety considerations. Both situations may limit dogs' natural behaviours as social animals and yet are so common that few may consider them to be poor welfare. Similarly, the nature of farming entails a delicate balance between oft-competing aims to maximize animal productivity, health and welfare while also accounting for economy, environmental impact, worker health and safety, and consumer interests. While improvements and change are attainable, compromise is likely inherent to their pursuit. Recognizing that some (animal) interests may be limited in order for animal-keeping to remain possible may to some degree unite animal owners in a common understanding that such measures are necessary if animals are to be safe, managed and living among us. Ultimately, accepting compromise may allow one to achieve perspective and bolster resilience when desired outcomes take more time or effort to realize, or when 100% compliance to the ideal vision cannot yet be reached.

4. *Cultivate openness and be prepared to acknowledge scientific uncertainty.* Animal welfare is a continuously evolving field and its practitioners must therefore

Continued

Continued.

practise continuous improvement of techniques. Yet animal practitioners often lack formal behaviour and welfare training (Rioja-Lang et al., 2020). This is especially problematic considering that those often framed as experts in matters of animal care may often lack training in *matters related to animal care*. Moreover, the prevalence of issues that remain underexplored or as of yet unanswered, compounded with the ethics that inform the very nature of animal welfare science, underscores the importance of acknowledging the limits of one's own advice or information. Public perspectives may in and of themselves be valuable in achieving progress as well, for example, by introducing new ways of thinking or new knowledge. Acknowledging the limitations of one's own knowledge and cultivating an openness to learning more may make communications more complicated, but also more objective (Sandøe et al., 2004) and hence valuable in achieving progress for animal welfare.

Acknowledgements

The authors are grateful to Dr Katy Proudfoot (Atlantic Veterinary College, University of Prince Edward Island) for her insight on an earlier version of this chapter.

References

Averós, X., Aparicio, M.A., Ferrari, P., Guy, J.H., Hubbard, C. et al. (2013) The effect of steps to promote higher levels of farm animal welfare across the EU. Societal versus animal scientists' perceptions of animal welfare. *Animals* 3(3), 786–807. doi:10.3390/ani3030786

Bell, E., Norwood, F.B. and Lusk, J.L. (2017) Are consumers wilfully ignorant about animal welfare? *Animal Welfare* 26(4), 399–402. doi:10.7120/09627286.26.4.399

Benard, M. and de Cock Buning, T. (2013) Exploring the potential of Dutch pig farmers and urban-citizens to learn through frame reflection. *Journal of Agricultural and Environmental Ethics* 26(5), 1015–1036. doi:10.1007/s10806-013-9438-y

Broom, D.M. (1991) Animal welfare: concepts and measurement. *Journal of Animal Science* 69, 4167–4175.

Buddle, E.A., Bray, H.J. and Ankeny, R.A. (2021) 'Of course we care!': A qualitative exploration of Australian producers' understandings of farm animal welfare issues. *Journal of Rural Studies* 83, 50–59. doi:10.1016/j.jrurstud.2021.02.024

Cummins, A., Olynk Widmar, N., Croney, C. and Fulton, J. (2015) *Perceptions of United States Residents: Animal Agriculture and Meat Products Executive Summary*. Center for Animal Welfare Science, Purdue University, West Lafayette, Indiana.

Duncan, I. (1993) Welfare is to do with what animals feel. *Journal of Agricultural and Environmental Ethics* 6(Suppl. 2), 8–14.

Ellis, K., Billington, K., McNeil, B. and McKeegan, D. (2009) Public opinion on UK milk marketing and dairy cow welfare. *Animal Welfare* 18(3), 267–282.

Eurobarometer 270 (2007) Attitudes of EU citizens towards animal welfare. Available at: https://ec.europa.eu/commfrontoffice/publicopinion/archives/ebs/ebs_270_en.pdf (accessed 18 July 2020).

Eurobarometer 442 (2016) Attitudes of Europeans towards animal welfare. Available at: https://ec.europa.eu/commfrontoffice/publicopinionmobile/index.cfm/Survey/getSurveyDetail/surveyKy/2096 (accessed 18 July 2020).

Evans, A.B. and Miele, M. (2019) Enacting public understandings: The case of farm animal welfare. *Geoforum* 99, 1–10. doi:10.1016/j.geoforum.2018.12.013

Fraser, D., Weary, D.M., Pajor, E.A. and Milligan, B.N. (1997) A scientific conception of animal welfare that reflects ethical concerns. *Animal Welfare* 6(3), 187–205.

García Pinillos, R. (2018) *One Welfare: A Framework to Improve Animal Welfare and Human Well-being*. CAB International, Wallingford, UK

Grigg, E.K. and Kogan, L.R. (2019) Owners' attitudes, knowledge, and care practices: Exploring the implications for domestic cat behavior and welfare in the home. *Animals* 9(978). doi:10.3390/ani9110978

Hansen, J., Holm, L., Frewer, L., Robinson, P. and Sandøe, P. (2003) Beyond the knowledge deficit: Recent research into lay and expert attitudes to food risks. *Appetite* 41, 111–121. doi:10.1016/S0195-6663(03)00079-5

Hecht, J., Miklósi, Á. and Gácsi, M. (2012) Behavioral assessment and owner perceptions of behaviors associated with guilt in dogs. *Applied Animal Behaviour Science* 139(1–2), 134–142. doi:10.1016/j.applanim.2012.02.015

Jacobs, J.A., Pearl, D., Coe, J., Widowski, T. and Niel, L. (2017) Ability of owners to identify resource guarding behaviour in the domestic dog. *Applied Animal Behaviour Science* 188, 77–83. doi:10.1016/j.applanim.2016.12.012

Kahneman, D. (2011) *Thinking Fast and Slow*. Farrar, Straus and Giroux, New York.

McDermott, M.P., Cobb, M.A., Tischler, V.A., Robbé, I.J. and Dean, R.S. (2017) Evaluating veterinary practitioner perceptions of communication skills and training. *Veterinary Record* 180(12), 305. doi:10.1136/vr.103997

McKendree, M.G.S., Croney, C.C. and Widmar, N.J.O. (2014) Effects of demographic factors and information sources on United States consumer perceptions of animal welfare. *Journal of Animal Science* 92(7), 3161–3173. doi:10.2527/jas.2014-6874

Mossop, L., Gray, C., Blaxter, A., Gardiner, A., MacEachern, K., Watson, P. et al. (2015) Communication skills training: What the vet schools are doing. *Veterinary Record* 176(5), 114–117. doi:10.1136/vr.h425

Nordengen, K. (2019) *Hjernen er stjernen (Your Superstar Brain: Unlocking the Secrets of the Human Mind)*. Kagge Forlag AS, Oslo.

Nyhan, B. and Reifler, J. (2010) When corrections fail: The persistence of political misperceptions. *Political Behavior* 32(2), 303–330. doi:10.1007/s11109-010-9112-2

Proudfoot, K. and Ventura, B. (2020) Impact of a frame reflection assignment on veterinary student perspectives toward animal welfare and difffering viewpoints. *Journal of Veterinary Medical Education*, e20190123. doi:10.3138/jvme.2019-0123

Rioja-Lang, F., Bacon, H., Connor, M. and Dwyer, C.M. (2020) Prioritisation of animal welfare issues in the UK using expert consensus. *Veterinary Record* 187(12), 490. doi:10.1136/vr.105964

Rollin, B. (1993) Animal welfare, science and value. *Journal of Agricultural and Environmental Ethics* 6(Suppl. 2), 44–50.

Ryan, E.B., Fraser, D. and Weary, D.M. (2015) Public attitudes to housing systems for pregnant pigs. *PLoS ONE* 10(11), e0141878. doi:10.1371/journal.pone.0141878.

Sandøe, P., Forkman, B. and Christiansen, S.B. (2004) Scientific uncertainty – How should it be handled in relation to scientific advice regarding animal welfare issues? *Animal Welfare* 13(Suppl.), S121–S126.

Schön, D.A. and Rein, M. (1994) *Frame Reflection: Toward the Resolution of Intractable Policy Controversies*. Basic Books, New York.

Serpell, J.A. (2019) How happy is your pet? The problem of subjectivity in the assessment of companion animal welfare. *Animal Welfare* 28(1), 57–66. doi:10.7120/09627286.28.1.057

Shaw, J.R. (2006) Four core communication skills of highly effective practitioners. *Veterinary Clinics of North America – Small Animal Practice* 36(2), 385–396. doi:10.1016/j.cvsm.2005.10.009

Simis, M.J., Madden, H., Cacciatore, M.A. and Yeo, S.K. (2016) The lure of rationality: Why does the deficit model persist in science communication? *Public Understanding of Science* 25(4), 400–414. doi:10.1177/0963662516629749

Vanhonacker, F., Verbeke, W., Poucke, E. and Tuyttens, F. (2007) Segmentation based on consumers' perceived importance and attitude toward farm animal welfare. *International Journal of Sociology of Food and Agriculture* 15(3), 84–100.

Ventura, B. (2015) Understanding industry and lay perspectives on dairy cattle welfare. Thesis, University of British Columbia.

Ventura, B.A., von Keyserlingk, M.A.G., Wittman, H. and Weary, D.M. (2016) What difference does a visit make? Changes in animal welfare perceptions after interested citizens tour a dairy farm. *PLoS ONE* 11(5), e0154733. doi:10.1371/journal.pone.0154733

Ventura, B., Terreaux, C. and Zhitnitskiy, P. (2020) Veterinary student knowledge and attitudes about swine change after lectures and a farm visit. *Journal of Veterinary Medical Education*, e20190160. doi:10.3138/jvme-2019-0160

Ventura, B., Weary, D. and von Keyserlingk, M. (n.d.) Ambivalence, resignation, and hope: European veterinarians' and researchers' views toward public concerns and roles in resolving challenges to cattle welfare. In preparation.

Verbeke, W. (2009) Stakeholder, citizen and consumer interests in farm animal welfare. *Animal Welfare* 18, 325–333.

Williams, L.A., Brosnan, S.F. and Clay, Z. (2020) Anthropomorphism in comparative affective science: Advocating a mindful approach. *Neuroscience and Biobehavioral Reviews* 115, 299–307. doi:10.1016/j.neubiorev.2020.05.014

Wood, T. and Porter, E. (2016) The elusive backfire effect: Mass attitudes' steadfast factual adherence. *Political Behavior* 41(1), 135–163. https://doi.org/10.1007/s11109-018-9443-y

Wynne, B. and Irwin, A. (1996) *Misunderstanding Science? The Public Reconstruction of Science and Technology*. Cambridge University Press, Cambridge, UK.

Ziv, G. (2017) The effects of using aversive training methods in dogs – A review. *Journal of Veterinary Behavior: Clinical Applications and Research* 19, 50–60. doi:10.1016/j.jveb.2017.02.004

It Takes a Village: Community Engagement for Sustainable Animal Welfare

4

Melissa Liszewski
International Fund for Animal Welfare (IFAW), London, UK

4.1 Introduction

There are billions of animals around the world whose welfare is impacted by the behaviour of individuals on a daily basis. The question of how to generate collective action to leverage change for animals at scale is no doubt burned into many of our brains. Collective action that leads to impact for populations of animals requires one key ingredient: community.

An unvaccinated dog abandoned on a rabies-endemic island in Indonesia, a farmer in Morocco struggling to protect crops from hungry endangered monkeys and a young donkey cart driver in Kenya striving to be seen as someone with a profession and a future. These real-life examples are both glaring proof of the direct links between animal welfare, human wellbeing and the environment and stark reminders that root causes not triggered solely by the actions of individuals cannot be solved at population level by employing individual approaches. External resources may help relieve immediate suffering caused by these problems, but relief will be short lived unless the people living closest to the animals and affected by the issues themselves collectively own and implement solutions that work for them.

In a world where economic inequalities, climate change, pandemics and myriad other threats face humans on a daily basis, how does one even begin to engage entire communities in animal welfare? This chapter is aimed at helping animal welfare practitioners do just that; laying out key principles, frameworks, practical guidance and real-life examples of community engagement for sustainable animal welfare.

4.1.1 Definitions of quality

Any animal welfare practitioner working in community engagement will be familiar with being told that their work sounds amazing, only to be immediately followed up with 'but what is it that you actually do?' Both 'community' and 'engagement' are vague enough terms on their own, let alone when placed together and in the context of animal welfare. Starting with definitions for commonly used terms and phrases in relation to community engagement, as they pertain to animal welfare, is a good place to begin (see Table 4.1).

Community engagement for animal welfare comes in all shapes and sizes and many different approaches can lead to success. There are some key standards that commonly signify quality community engagement however (adapted from the United Nations International Children's Emergency Fund's (UNICEF) Minimum Quality Standards and Indicators for Community Engagement, 2020).

1. *Participation*: What needs to be done, how it should be done and what success looks like is identified, prioritized and planned with community members and integrated into the initiative, with efforts made to reduce barriers to participation throughout planning and implementation.
- Every community has assets, knowledge, and potential for development and leadership. Rarely is it truly the case that an external person or group must feed, treat or shelter all animals in need because the community themselves can't or won't. The role of a community facilitator is to help them harness their available resources to reach their goals in a way they can sustain after the external engagement and support ends.
- In Morocco, where dozens of fruit farms with adjacent properties were each paying guards – if it was affordable to them – to chase monkeys away from their own crops, the community was supported to come together for the first time to discuss this shared challenge and form an official community association for sharing information and community resources (e.g. trained community guards rather than untrained individual guards) to mitigate crop raiding more efficiently and effectively (see Case Study 2).

Table 4.1. Community engagement definitions.

Term	Definition
Community engagement	A strategic process by which an individual or organization builds relationships and partnerships with groups of people for the purpose of applying a collective vision that benefits animals and people
Community	Groupings of individuals sharing a geographic location, practice, interest or circumstance that relates to or impacts on animals
Community facilitator	A person who helps a community work together, define shared goals and plan how to achieve those goals to benefit animals and people
Sustainability	The degree to which impacts for animals and their communities are able to be maintained over time in a given setting, particularly after exit of external support

2. *Empowerment and ownership*: Community members feel they own the initiative(s) and that they are in fact for them and not simply to satisfy external organizations or donors, with capacity-building measures to strengthen community leadership built in as needed.
- If external actors lead in every aspect of a community animal welfare initiative without working every day as though they are trying to make their roles redundant by the end of the engagement, they risk creating dependencies on external actors to provide band-aid fixes that may be ripped off as soon as funding runs out, or the organization shifts priorities.
- In Indonesia, when a non-governmental organization (NGO)-led community-based rabies and dog welfare initiative neared the end of its project cycle, local leaders in three communities were so proud of and invested in the improvements they saw that they agreed to integrate support to continue activities after the end of the project into their own annual village budgets.

3. *Inclusion*: All members of the community are included in activities, decision making and access to services, with efforts made to ensure voices of disadvantaged and marginalized individuals or social groups are sought out and amplified.
- Identifying and involving the people and stakeholders affected by the focus of the engagement is an important but all too easily overlooked component of quality community engagement. It is not a given that all stakeholders naturally have the opportunity to participate in decisions that affect them within their community so extra steps must be taken to ensure that everyone who wants to be and should be included has every opportunity to do so (see Fig. 4.1).
- In India, after several engagements with male equine owners it became clear that many of the husbandry changes needing to be made were the responsibility of women in the community, although to date they had not been able to directly access the information and resources provided. Women's equine welfare groups were developed so they could not only access information and resources, but start group savings to facilitate access to animal health services, education or emergency household needs (see Fig. 4.2).

4. *Two-way communication*: Information is clearly and consistently provided to communities throughout the engagement process and a mechanism is in place to enable them to give regular feedback that ensures their experience, views and concerns are incorporated.
- Every interaction with a community is an opportunity for learning and understanding how animal welfare initiatives can best suit their needs and interests. It's also an opportunity to share results from recent data collection, or inform them of news or activities with other stakeholders that may affect them. Expectations should be carefully managed every step of the way to avoid loss of trust or disappointment. If building a vet clinic is something they want but is unlikely to be delivered, this should be clarified early and often while trying to better understand the core of what they really need. If it's closer and easier access to quality animal health services, there are many other ways to help them achieve this that do not require ongoing building management, maintenance and equipment support.

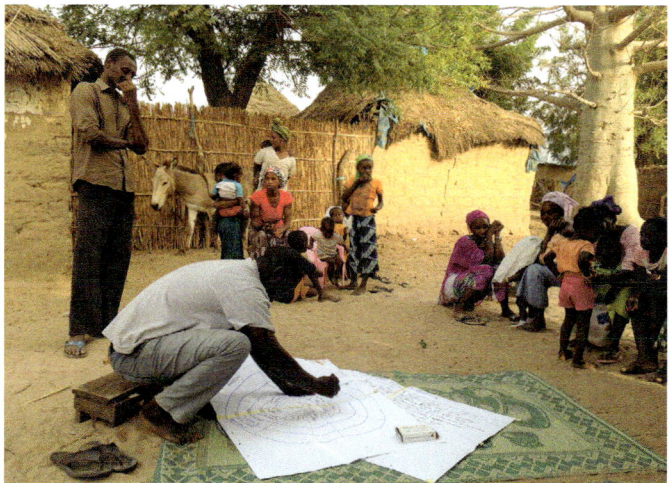

Fig. 4.1. Analysing gender roles as they relate to animals in Senegal.

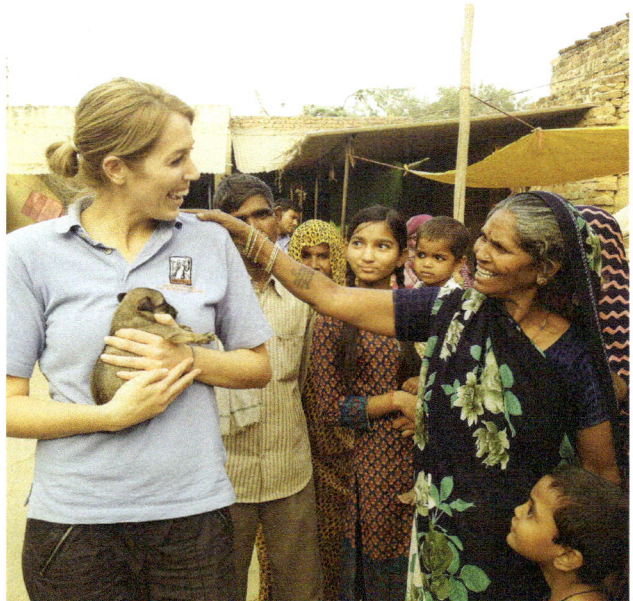

Fig. 4.2. Author Melissa at a women's group meeting in India.

- In a community meeting in Kenya, where its donkey owners were previously assumed not to be using newly improved veterinary services because of the cost, an open facilitated discussion between them and the vets revealed the true reason to be that they felt the vets did not treat them with enough respect. This learning enabled the project to develop activities far better suited to the true barrier to change than would have otherwise been pursued without effective communication, such as increased linkage meetings between local animal healthcare providers and communities to strengthen relationships.

5. *Adaptability and localization*: Approaches and activities are continuously tailored to suit local needs, resources and realities guided by stakeholders who know the context best, with plans adapted based on community feedback and data (see Fig. 4.3).
- Context is everything when it comes to community engagement. Trying to achieve standards completely outside of local customs and systems, or introducing animal husbandry tools and services not locally available or accessible, risks demotivating communities and sending a message that animal welfare is out of their reach. Having a solid understanding of barriers they face, such as whether they have the capability (e.g. knowledge and skills), motivation (e.g. willingness, enthusiasm) and opportunity (e.g. resources, enabling environment) (Michie *et al.*, 2011) to make the required animal welfare changes is a useful place to start (see Case Study 1).
- In rural Ethiopia, where donkeys were suffering from external parasites and poor hoof health, and hoof picks and curry combs are not widely available, owners were encouraged to use a stick or metal spoon to clean hooves and shown how to make curry combs out of metal bottle caps nailed to a block of wood (see Fig. 4.4).

6. *Building on local capacity*: Animal welfare initiatives are integrated into existing community systems, structures and services wherever possible, with an aim to strengthen and build upon what already exists prior to creating something completely new. Bolstering governance, social accountability and

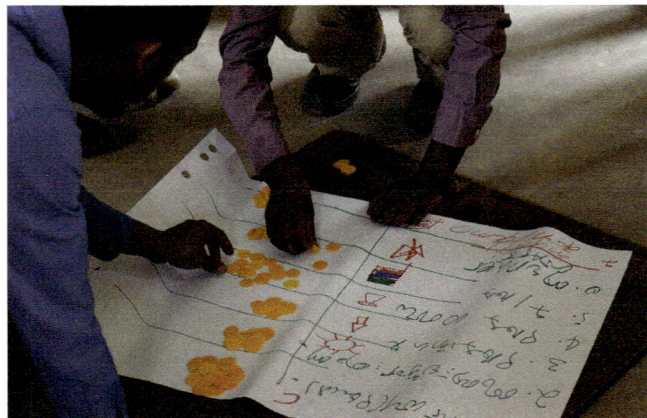

Fig. 4.3. Animal owners using an assessment method accessible to the whole group in Ethiopia.

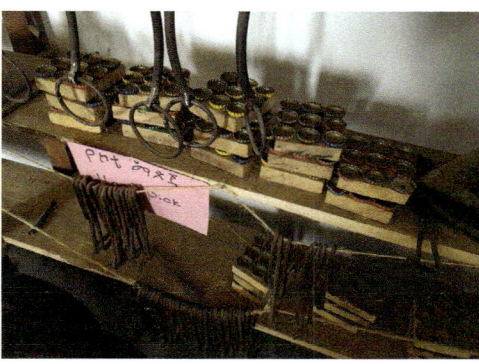

Fig. 4.4. Locally made husbandry tools in Ethiopia.

economic opportunities of community-based organizations (CBOs) or community-based enterprises (CBEs) is prioritized to ensure sustainable local capacity for collective action.

- Even if not obvious at first glance, there are opportunities in every community to build upon existing skills and resources already present for years, if not generations, within the community. If local people don't have the right skills or equipment, it will do little to help animals and people in the long run if external experts are brought in to do the job without any concurrent efforts to build community capacity.
- In rural Ethiopia where government-run Farmer Training Centres (i.e. agricultural extension services) were already available in donkey-owning communities, an equine welfare curriculum aimed at addressing the top welfare issues in the local donkey population were integrated into the curriculum and development agents responsible for delivering content were trained in equine welfare.

Participatory, community leadership and respecting local knowledge by no means discount the value that technical experts bring to specific aspects of any community engagement project, especially when it comes to animal welfare. There is a time and place for technical animal health or welfare advice to be provided during every project, but rarely should this be the primary or only purpose of a community initiative. Where external capacity must be brought in to advise on specific issues or services, there should always be an attempt to leave that knowledge and expertise with a professional in the community, so the skills and services remain even after the NGO or other external project initiator leaves.

4.2 Strategic Engagement

A common misconception in the NGO world is that a community is simply 'the people we work with' (Titz *et al.*, 2018), but communities are not homogeneous so there will always be a variety of subgroups, experiences, interests and abilities to consider. It is often unnecessary and impractical to work with the entire community or tailor engagement to every individual within it, so community engagement needs to be strategic in order to ensure the desired results for animals.

As a first step towards strategic engagement, the target individuals and group(s) able to directly contribute to key welfare issues need to be identified and understood. This can be done by analysing the role and perspective of different subgroups within a community in relation to their potential contribution to the key welfare issues. Following this step, the most effective way to engage will become clearer after spending some time chatting with a diverse range of individuals representing them to understand the characteristics, relationships, diversity and power structures that may influence their ability to address welfare issues. Whenever possible, working with a local community facilitator who already knows the culture, community dynamics and potential entry points will allow the work to progress more quickly and effectively, while embedding local leadership from the start.

Take for example a town in Nicaragua with carriage horses experiencing heat stress on a regular basis. An immediate and well-intentioned reaction would probably be to engage carriage drivers in heat stress prevention training and provide them with free buckets to keep in carriages to facilitate water provision or cool down sessions for animals during the workday. Although seemingly straightforward enough, after digging a bit deeper a local NGO team learned that shop owners unfairly charged carriage drivers to fill water buckets, local police fined carriage drivers when horses urinated on the town's historic cobblestone streets, owner's wives played a significant role in feeding and watering practices, and a number of carriage drivers rented rather than owned their horse, so had less incentive to invest in welfare improvements. A change in carriage driver behaviour – regardless of owner or renter status – would bring significant welfare improvements; however, the only way to achieve that was by widening engagement beyond the individuals directly responsible for making the changes sought and focusing on reducing barriers those key stakeholders faced to implementing change.

4.3 Characterizing Communities

Although understanding key characteristics of a target community is critical to developing an effective engagement strategy, it can be a complex and intensive process that many teams do not have the time to pursue prior to developing their plans. At a minimum, it is helpful for practitioners to: (i) clarify the purpose that brings their target community together, and (ii) understand the stability of membership and (iii) the level of social cohesion (see Table 4.2). A note of caution however: characterizing communities is not meant to label or judge them and is in no way indicative of the worth of the community or what its members are capable of achieving. It is merely a useful guide to help

Table 4.2. Characterizing communities.

Purpose	Stability	Social cohesion
Practice-based Network of people with specialized interest, expertise or professional experience that exchange information, work together, imagine a shared identity and/or align their activities towards a shared goal (Räsänen et al., 2020)	**Stable** Generally low turnover, with the same members remaining for a long period of time even if leadership and other structural changes occur more frequently. For example, non-migratory brick kiln where people and animals live at the site year-round	**Strong** High levels of unity, commonality and agreement. Group socialization or working through shared problems or projects is not uncommon. Active community initiatives may already be present and generally function well, bringing benefits back into the community
Place-based[a] Individuals bound together by the geographical location in which they live, work and spend free time. Includes all individuals and social structures in a geographical location such as inhabitants, organizations, institutions and authorities	**Mixed** Significant member turnover on a regular basis but a core group remains over time or regularly moves away for a period but always returns. For example, brick kiln where some people and animals migrate to a site for the season while others are permanent residents/workers	**Medium** Unity, commonality and agreement can be found in subsets of the community but some disagreement exists between subsets. Socializing in groups and working together may happen in factions, but only benefits individuals and/or subsets of the community
Circumstance Communities of people brought together by external events/situations, interactions, shared life experiences or identity	**Dynamic** High turnover of members with individuals regularly moving in/out or only staying for short periods of time. For example, brick kiln where people and animals migrate to a site for a working season and then disperse to their permanent homes at the end without returning to the same site the following year	**Weak** Individualism, disagreement and resistance among members is common. Socializing in groups, helping each other and working towards shared goals or through shared problems is not common. Active social groups and community initiatives are not present or functioning in a way that benefits the community

[a] Further characterizing as urban, peri-urban or rural is often helpful as this will significantly impact the strategy required.

practitioners realistically estimate the length, type and depth of engagement that may be required to achieve their animal welfare goals.

Communities do not operate in a bubble however, but within complex networks and broader systems including government, NGOs, service providers, businesses and a variety of other stakeholders. So while the majority of time at the beginning of a community engagement initiative will likely be dedicated to getting to know the target community themselves, developing a better understanding of the entire local animal welfare system over time will better ensure a holistic engagement strategy. Whether linking target communities with others to help them achieve their goals, advocating for them to be listened to or building capacity of others to better meet their needs, secondary individuals and groups needing to be integrated into the engagement strategy will emerge as work progresses.

4.4 Characterizing Engagement

When developing a community engagement strategy, clarifying the type of approach best suited to the target group(s) and severity and prevalence of welfare issues will guide a realistic appraisal of time and resource requirements. For ongoing initiatives this can be done by reviewing existing depth and breadth of participation (Farrington *et al.* cited in Cornwall, 2008) and intensity of engagement alongside welfare results achieved, to identify gaps that could make the engagement more effective or impact more sustainable. Ideally this type of review is always done together with the community.

While the depth of participation refers to how engaged participants are in all stages of an animal welfare initiative, from inception through to implementation and reflection, breadth refers to the range of people participating. Engagement may be narrow, for example, if only male farmers participate, but deep if those individuals are actively involved in every stage of the process. Few animal welfare organizations have the time and resources to achieve both high depth and wide breadth, which is why careful selection of the specific groups of individuals within a community that need to be targeted is crucial.

Intensity could be a simpler and more useful metric for community-based animal welfare work as it refers holistically to the depth, breadth and frequency of engagement (see Table 4.3), with an intensive approach generally necessary to address widespread, deeply rooted or severe welfare issues. Conversely, an extensive engagement approach is often useful in scenarios where welfare issues are less prevalent, severe or deeply rooted; these approaches can also be effective in communities where a strong animal welfare foundation already exists and new initiatives are more likely to be taken up easily and quickly.

There is a time and place for every level and type of community engagement depending on what you're trying to achieve in the long run. It may not be appropriate, desirable or necessary for every community to lead and manage every animal welfare initiative themselves so although community empowerment is the highest level to ensure local ownership and sustainability (see Table 4.4) it may not be the gold standard for every scenario. What matters most is striving to achieve optimum participation for the target communities, meaning the right balance of depth, breadth and frequency for the purpose of the initiative (Cornwall, 2008).

Table 4.3. Characterizing engagement.

Intensive engagement	Extensive engagement
Relatively high frequency of engagement with the same individuals, focused on achieving high depth of participation but often only able to reach narrow breadth with a few targeted groups of actors	Relatively low frequency of engagement with the same individuals, focused on achieving low depth of participation but often able to reach wider breadth across the whole community
Examples: supporting formation of a community committee to deal with abandoned animals or human wildlife conflict, or a cart and harness improvement project engaging owners, local artisans and service providers bi-weekly	Examples: an initiative to reduce feeding monkeys at a popular tourist site, or an annual campaign focused on conveying the why/when/where of government-administered rabies vaccines in a village

Table 4.4. Levels of engagement.

Empower
Community leads in all aspects of deciding and acting on what needs to be done to improve animal welfare; external actors provide only facilitation and technical support and minimal financial, material and service support

Collaborate
Community is treated as an equal partner where joint decision making and action related to animal welfare initiatives occur throughout each aspect of the project

Involve
Community is asked about their needs and preferences with regards to animal welfare and these are incorporated into the plan, with progress reported back to them throughout the process

Consult
Community is asked for feedback on what should be done about animal welfare issues, the quality and effectiveness of services and/or activities being offered but not otherwise involved

Inform
Community is provided with information on animal welfare issues, services being offered or activities being implemented but not consulted

Intensity of engagement
Level of community leadership
Facilitation skills required

Level headings from IAP2 Spectrum of Public Participation (2018).

Case Study 1: Strategic Application of a Behaviour Change Model

With over 11 million equids in Ethiopia (FAO, 2018), most of which are involved in transport of commodities and people, working animals are a daily lifeline to countless families around the country. Alaba Kulito is an important market and communication town (kulito) in the Southern Nations, Nationalities, and Peoples' Region (SNNPR) of Ethiopia (Alaba Kulito, 2020). Inadequate social infrastructure, underdeveloped public services and poverty are predominant challenges facing this rapidly growing urban area. Despite the critical importance of Alaba's >3000 working equids, they suffer from high prevalence and severity of wounds, lameness and hoof issues, poor handling, overworking, eye problems, inadequate resting areas and abandonment. A 2013 welfare assessment revealed that 70% of gharry (taxi) horses had a highly compromised ability to walk and nearly 70% of owners surveyed were not providing quality shelter for animals to rest in (unpublished, Brooke, 2013).

A local team from Brooke – an international charity working to improve the lives of horses, donkeys and mules – tried for several years to engage gharry owners in the town but found it difficult to do so in a way that was effective and sustainable. Challenges the team faced included lacklustre response to capacity-building activities, high turnover of animals, low welfare motivation of operators renting horses,

Capability	Motivation
Gharry owners have the knowledge, skills and physical ability to improve welfare practices	*Gharry owners have the desire, enthusiasm and inspiration to improve welfare practices*
Key barriers: Inconsistent knowledge of animal welfare and husbandry practices Poor understanding of importance of quality animal health services Unaware of severity and impact of welfare issues affecting animal(s)	**Key barriers:** Feeling alone, unsupported and unable to make changes Lack of perceived benefit due to dynamic and competing priorities Inadequate local regulations to support animal welfare initiatives
Interventions: • Bi-weekly meetings with equine owners to discuss priority welfare issues, causes and solutions • Training manual for community facilitators to ensure technical understanding of priority welfare issues • Training and demonstration sessions for owners and service providers • Joint welfare appraisals with owners and sharing standardized welfare assessment data • Raise awareness on euthanasia rather than abandonment	**Interventions:** • 1 to 1 support and encouragement to provide personalized help to owners at home • Incentives such as free feed for best improvements made • Local by-law improvement to safeguard against intentional harm • Integrated welfare and livelihoods messaging • Local veterinary, farriery and husbandry services integrated into equine shelter for easier and quicker access • Collaboration of local committees to monitor neighbourhoods for abandoned animals

Opportunity

Gharry owners have an enabling and encouraging environment

Key barriers:
Lack of affordable, accessible and quality animal health services
Limited affordable, accessible and quality husbandry resources
Inadequate system for support and collaboration

Interventions:
• Linkage meetings with local officials, gharry owners and animal health providers to build collaboration
• Improve availability, affordability and accessibility of feed, water and husbandry equipment
• Capacity building of local vets, farriers and Gharry Horse Owners Association
• Expand operation of equine welfare centre and hand over to Gharry Horse Owners Association

Fig. 4.5. Adapting strategy to reduce barriers

Continued

> **Case Study 1:** Continued
>
> poor enforcement of driver's licence requirements and a lack of accessible quality health and husbandry services, leading to owners spending upwards of 30% of their daily income caring for their horse. In 2014, the project team began testing a new method to sustainably engage and motivate local stakeholders that focused on addressing key barriers gharry owners faced in making welfare improvements for their animals. Interventions were balanced to equally address the three key factors needing to be present for any behaviour to occur, as laid out by the COM-B model of behaviour (Michie *et al.*, 2011) (see Fig. 4.5).
>
> Despite an initially modest goal of engaging just 30 motivated owners in a single kebele (neighbourhood) out of the estimated 700–1000 spread across 79 kebeles, the team managed to achieve genuine engagement of over 250 owners in the first 6 months. At the end of the pilot participants themselves suggested they be trained as community change agents to work through existing structures to transfer knowledge more widely and motivate fellow owners within and outside of their kebele. In addition to contributing to animal welfare gains in Alaba Kulito, human wellbeing benefited from increased access to information, resources and peer support to strengthen resilience of equine-based livelihoods.
>
> Case study adapted from Liszewski (2017)

4.5 The Engagement Process

Every community and context is different so there is no recipe to follow for engagement that guarantees success every single time, but any initiative without a clearly defined plan risks veering off track and trying to do too much, especially one as complex as a participatory community initiative. When this happens, even with the best of intentions, there is risk of harming the very animals and people animal welfare practitioners are trying to help by making them dependent on external – and ultimately temporary – people to meet their needs. There are countless more animals and people around the world who could also use a little help but may never receive it if practitioners are only ever able to work in a small handful of communities without exiting.

This is exactly why community engagement by NGOs and other external actors should generally be treated as a project, which according to the Project Management Institute is 'a temporary endeavor undertaken to create a unique project service or result' with five key phases: initiation, planning, execution, monitoring and closure (PMI, 2008, p. 434). A community project can easily turn into a chicken-and-egg scenario however, when resources are required to initiate and plan in a participatory way, but project sponsors or donors require submission of a detailed plan and budget prior to granting any resources. Practitioners can find a happy middle ground being guided by a process that is systematic enough to provide a clear roadmap and reassure project sponsors there is a plan, but that remains flexible for the community to decide specifically what they want to do, how they want to do it and what success will look like.

The process that follows (see Fig. 4.6) is based on the author's experience of supporting and managing a variety of community projects in over

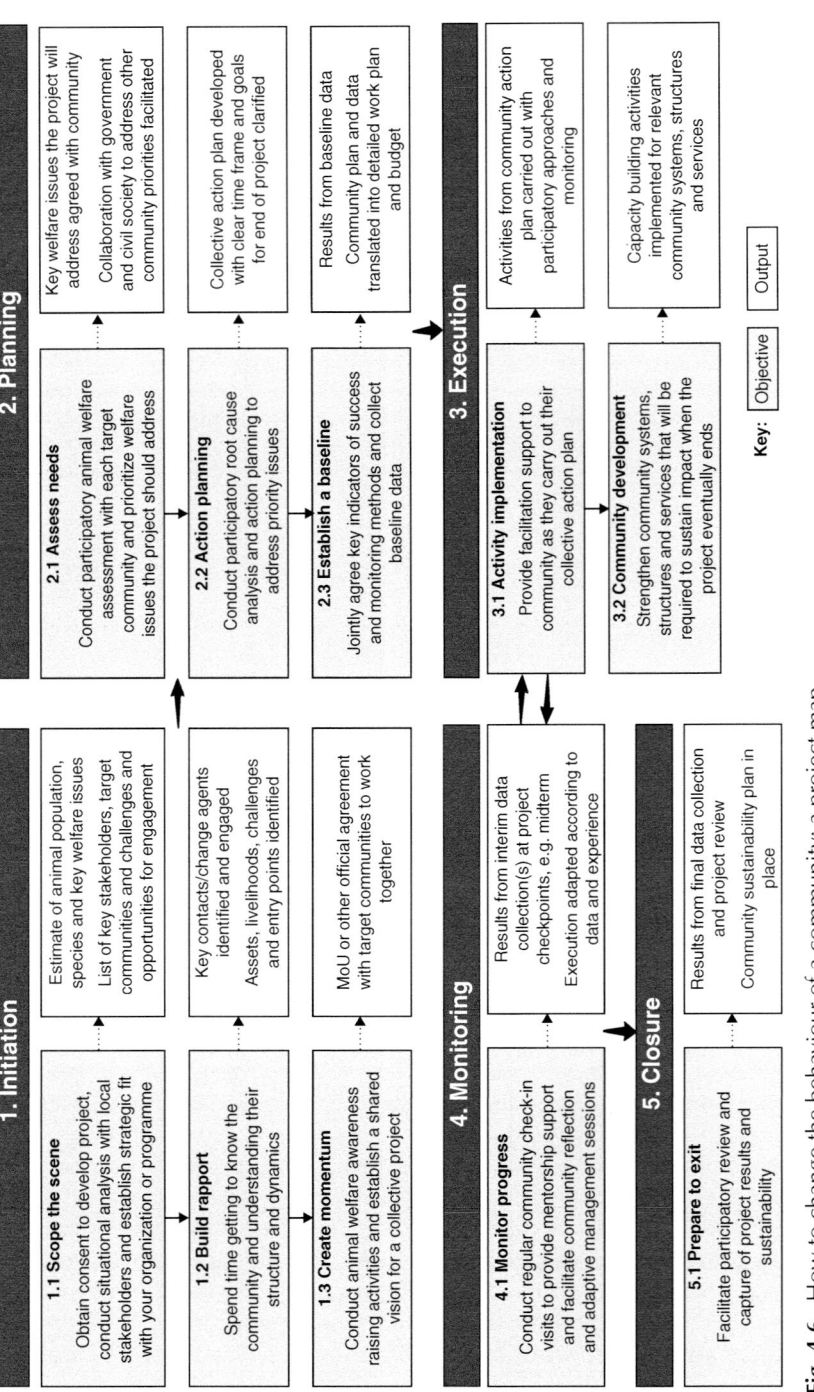

Fig. 4.6. How to change the behaviour of a community: a project map.

30 countries around the world and may serve as a helpful compass for animal welfare practitioners. Stages can and often do overlap or happen simultaneously and depending on the community, funding cycle, or the nature of welfare issues, a project may require additional steps not listed here. Therefore, you should not feel your project is wrong if your roadmap looks different.

> **Case Study 2: Deciding Where to Start in Morocco**
>
> Owing to habitat loss and poaching for the exotic pet trade, Barbary macaques are endangered animals and have been listed on CITES Appendix I (see Fig. 4.7). They are facing increasing threats in one of their last remaining natural habitats in Ifrane National Park in Morocco, where more than half of the surviving population is estimated to live (Ménard *et al.*, 2014). Born to be Wild is a project aimed at stopping the poaching and smuggling of Barbary macaques, strengthening enforcement capacity, and engaging local communities and tourists to ensure the welfare and conservation of these animals. Funded by the Dutch Postcode Lottery, the project was initiated by Animal Advocacy and Protection (AAP) and executed together with IFAW.
>
> Communities living near Ifrane National Park that rely on small-scale fruit and nut farming as a key part of their livelihood strategies have reported greatly increased crop-raiding activities by Barbary macaques and subsequent human–wildlife conflict in recent years. This is extremely detrimental to affected families, as lost crops not only reduce current yield but also damage and kill trees, thereby reducing future yields. This also threatens the welfare and conservation of Barbary macaques, as people may be tempted to retaliate and are less likely to support conservation initiatives if the species is considered a pest. Additionally, future reintroduction efforts of animals rescued from the exotic pet trade could be threatened without having a successful model for local human–animal coexistence in place.
>
> Out of countless communities living on the edge of the national park, however, the key question was where to start. In October 2018 more than 50 individuals from a community on the edge of the park wrote a joint letter to the governor about the crop-raiding issue they were having at their farms. Born to be Wild
>
>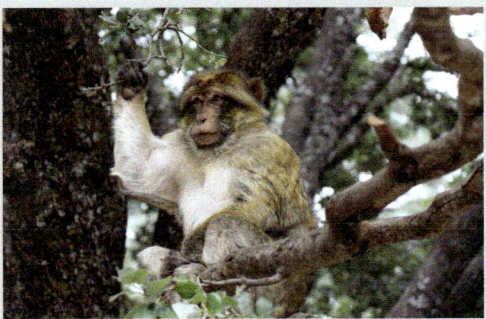
>
> **Fig. 4.7.** Barbary macaque in Ifrane National Park, Morocco. (© IFAW/Kinda Jabi.)

Continued

Case Study 2: Continued.

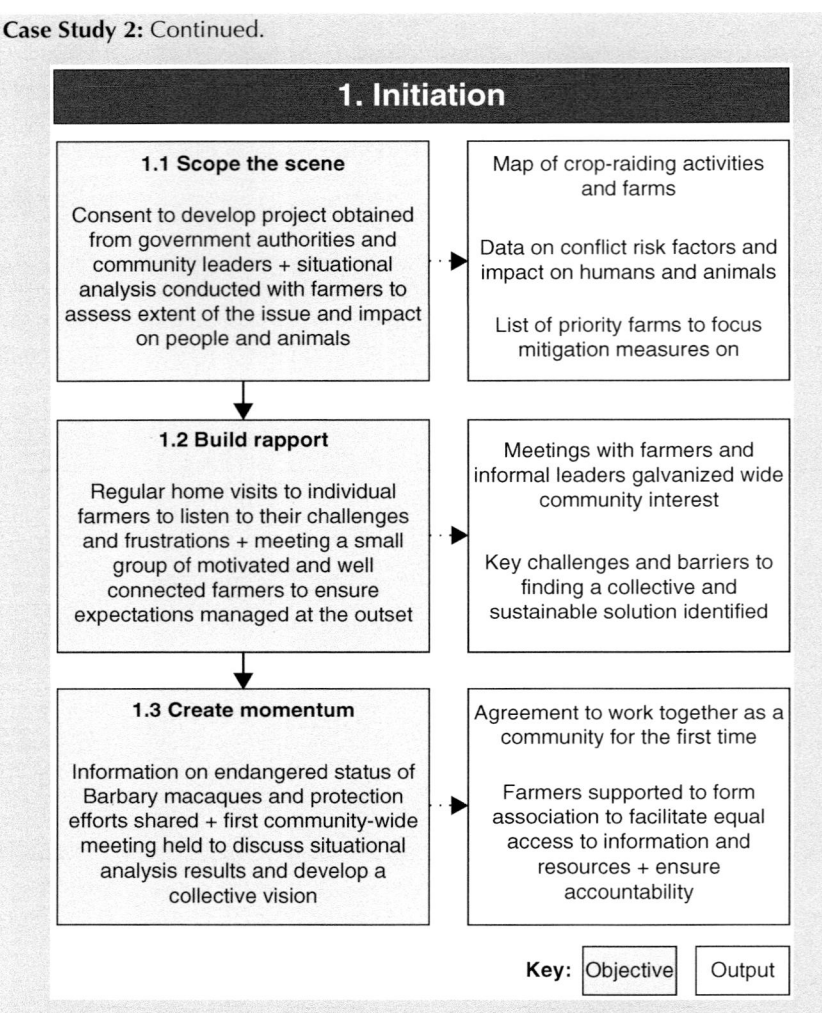

Fig. 4.8. How to initiate a community animal welfare project.

anti-poaching scouts had previously visited this community on a few occasions as part of their regular surveillance and awareness-raising work so the fit seemed right for project development. Initial expectations in the community were that financial compensation could be provided by the Born to be Wild project to offset losses owing to crop-raiding activities; however, this would not solve the problem or be able to be sustained after the end of the project. Thus, with the approval of the Water and Forests Department in Morocco, a project was initiated to help the community find a solution to this problem that they could sustain on their own and that could be replicated in future to help other communities in the region also facing this challenge (see Fig. 4.8).

4.6 Future Outlook

Aside from the animal and human impact of deeply engaging communities in animal welfare initiatives, quality engagement has the capability to inform decision making at a higher level, build capacity and strengthen relationships (Capire Consulting Group, 2016) critical to achieving systemic change for animal welfare. 'The first and most fundamental driver for systems change should be meeting the needs of [those benefiting from the system] and understanding the assets they have that can help' (Abercrombie *et al.*, 2015, p. 28). This places community engagement at the very heart of the wider systemic change required to address some of the world's most pressing animal welfare challenges and reinforces the ever-increasing need for skilled animal welfare practitioners in the profession.

There is no shortage of existing tools and techniques to aid animal welfare practitioners in implementing community engagement initiatives of all shapes and sizes; however, they will only ever be as effective as the facilitator applying them. Being a community facilitator is a professional discipline requiring specialized skills and the right personality and demeanour that not every individual has, or is able to be trained in. Further training in this is recommended, as described in Chapter 3, for the right individuals. They must be empathetic, observant, friendly, energetic, open-minded, patient and organized. While it can be helpful if they have technical expertise on the animals or welfare issues at hand, it is not entirely necessary. A good facilitator will always be astute enough to recognize when a challenge or opportunity requiring specialist knowledge is identified and will engage the right technical expert at the right time. New practitioners may find the best place to start is to enrol in a professional facilitation training course and practice tools and techniques tailor-made for application to animal welfare, such as Brooke's *Sharing the Load* (van Dijk *et al.*, 2011) or IFAW's Humane Community Development e-Learning (2019).

Even under the most challenging circumstances with some of the most severe welfare problems, change for animals and people is lurking just beneath the surface in every community, waiting for the right conditions and support to surface and transform the status quo. All animal welfare practitioners, whether working with individuals, businesses or governments, should be encouraged to try including community engagement in their work. They may be surprised at what they learn about the realities of caring for and living with animals that enriches and strengthens the work they are carrying out in unexpected but brilliant ways.

Acknowledgements

Thank you to Syed Naeem Abbas from Brooke Pakistan for his review of this chapter.

References

Abercrombie, R., Harries, E. and Wharton, R. (2015) Systems Change, a Guide to What it is and How to Do it. New Philanthropy Capital (NPC). Available at: https://www.thinknpc.org/resource-hub/systems-change-a-guide-to-what-it-is-and-how-to-do-it (accessed 10 September 2020).

Alaba Kulito (2020) Alaba Kulito. Wikipedia. Available at: https://en.wikipedia.org/wiki/Alaba_Kulito (accessed 10 September 2020).

Capire Consulting Group (2016) Inclusive Community Engagement Toolkit: version 2. Capire Consulting Group, Melbourne, Australia. Available at: https://www.tamarackcommunity.ca/hubfs/Resources/Tools/Capire%20Triangle%20Booklet.pdf (accessed 10 September 2020).

Cornwall, A. (2008) Unpacking 'participation' models, meanings and practices. *Community Development Journal* 43(3), 269–283.

Food and Agriculture Organization of the United Nations (FAO) (2018) FAOSTAT statistical database. FAO, Rome.

International Association for Public Participation (IAP2) (2018) The IAP2 public participation spectrum. Available at: https://cdn.ymaws.com/www.iap2.org/resource/resmgr/pillars/Spectrum_8.5x11_Print.pdf (accessed 9 September 2020).

International Fund for Animal Welfare (IFAW) (2019) Humane Community Development eLearning. International Companion Animal Management Coalition (ICAM). Available at: https://www.icam-coalition.org/tool/humane-community-development-hcd (accessed 31 March 2021).

Liszewski, M. (2017) Case study 2: Putting theory into practice in Halaba, Ethiopia. Exploring key HBC frameworks and principles. London, 17 May 2017 (unpublished).

Ménard, N., Rantier, Y., Foulquier, A., Qarro, M., Chillasse, L., Vallet, D. and Butet, A. (2014) Impact of human pressure and forest fragmentation on the endangered Barbary macaque *Macaca sylvanus* in the Middle Atlas of Morocco. *Oryx* 48(2), 276–284.

Michie, S., van Stralen, M.M. and West, R. (2011) The behaviour change wheel: A new method for characterising and designing behaviour change interventions. *Implementation Science* 6, 42.

Project Management Institute (PMI) (2008) A guide to the project management body of knowledge (PMBOK® guide), 4th edn. PMI, Newtown Square, Pennsylvania.

Räsänen, A., Lein, H., Bird, D. and Setten, G. (2020) Conceptualizing community in disaster risk management. *International Journal of Disaster Risk Reduction* 45, 101485.

Titz, A., Cannon, T. and Kruger, F. (2018) Uncovering 'community': Challenging an elusive concept in development and disaster related work. *Societies* 8(71), 1–28.

UNICEF (2020) Minimum quality standards and indicators in community engagement. Available at: https://www.unicef.org/mena/media/8401/file/19218_MinimumQuality-Report_v07_RC_002.pdf.pdf (accessed 9 September 2020).

van Dijk, L., Pritchard, J.C., Pradhan, S.K. and Wells, K. (2011) *Sharing the Load, a Guide to Improving the Welfare of Working Animals Through Collective Action*. Practical Action Publishing, Rugby, UK.

Educating the Animal Welfare Practitioners of the Future

5

Cathy Dwyer[1,2], Heather Bacon[1], Tamsin Coombs[2] and Fritha Langford[2]

[1]*The Royal (Dick) School of Veterinary Studies, University of Edinburgh, Edinburgh, UK;* [2]*Scotland's Rural College (SRUC), Edinburgh, UK*

5.1 Introduction

Education and awareness raising have played a pivotal role in increasing societal concern for the lives of non-human animals. Over the past 60 years or so there has been an increasing body of scientific research, which has asked questions about what animals need for good welfare, and quantified the impact on the animal of not having its needs or requirements met. The increasing science base means that our understanding of the welfare impact of various husbandry and management practices is growing. Where we need to construct arguments for changes in practice that may run counter to cultural or habitual norms, our knowledge of the science can be very important in demonstrating measurable animal welfare benefits. Education should cover animal welfare science and an understanding of different ethical viewpoints, as well as addressing why people make choices or behave in ways that may not seem rational or appropriate to ourselves. Understanding science and human decision making, and how behaviour is influenced, are crucial in improving animal welfare.

Animal welfare practitioners, who must navigate these complex arenas, require a scientific understanding of animal wants and needs, and an ability to carry out ethical reasoning and to advocate for animal welfare in legal and policy decisions. This requires education of veterinarians and other animal welfare professionals to have the skills to meet these complex requirements (De Briyne *et al.*, 2020).

5.2 Education, Beliefs and Attitudes

Who needs education in animal welfare? As animal welfare is identified as a societal concern, or everyone's responsibility, the short answer might be:

everyone. With this in mind educational programmes have been designed for many different groups including children, farmers, animal keepers, animal scientists and veterinarians (Coleman *et al.*, 2000; Illmann *et al.*, 2014; Lakestani *et al.*, 2015). Animal welfare education is particularly important for veterinarians, as they are frequently perceived (by themselves and others) as the 'leading advocates for the good welfare of animals' (FVE), and best placed to effect animal welfare change through educating their clients (Johnstone *et al.*, 2019). However, in many countries, animal welfare education for veterinarians is still in its infancy or entirely absent, and practical animal welfare activities are often carried out by industry, non-governmental organizations (NGOs) or government officials who have not had veterinary training. Animal welfare education is therefore also very relevant to animal scientists, who provide advice and consultancy to keepers of farm animals, and to advisers in a number of different roles that can impact on animal lives. This can be directly, through the actions of NGOs working with animal keepers, and indirectly through policy making in government and elsewhere.

Education is not just the act of learning and teaching in a school or college, but also the provision of an inspiring environment to facilitate learning, challenging bias and preconceptions, and recognizing that education can be achieved by means other than formal classroom-based teaching. In the past, most education was taught by traditional means – students were passive listeners and observers of their instructors, and most university education was of a lecture-based format. More recently though, it has become apparent that this is not as effective as other methods, particularly for a subject like animal welfare, which bridges the gap between science and ethics (Fraser *et al.*, 1997). Education that promotes discussion, thinking, debate, problem-based learning and methods that encourage the student to engage with the topic themselves is very important. For those working in animal welfare, these approaches provide students with the tools to acquire and assimilate new knowledge once they leave a formal education setting, rather than attempting to pass on all the current knowledge, much of which will become outdated and obsolete with time. This 'just in time' learning empowers students with the skills to find information needed at a particular time throughout their career, rather than memorizing enormous amounts of information 'just in case' (May and Silva-Fletcher, 2015). Because animal welfare can be a contested issue, advocacy skills such as learning to listen, debate and organize a coherent argument are as important as acquiring underpinning knowledge in bringing about improvements in animal welfare. Coleman (2010) suggests that the approach of providing targeted dispassionate and factual information to the community and actors where a change is required is most likely to produce good outcomes, as discussions are based on a shared understanding of current practice and scientific knowledge (Fig. 5.1).

Lack of knowledge, for example of the behavioural or other welfare needs of a species, is often identified as a welfare concern (Rioja-Lang *et al.*, 2020), and it is clear that targeted educational interventions can increase level of knowledge

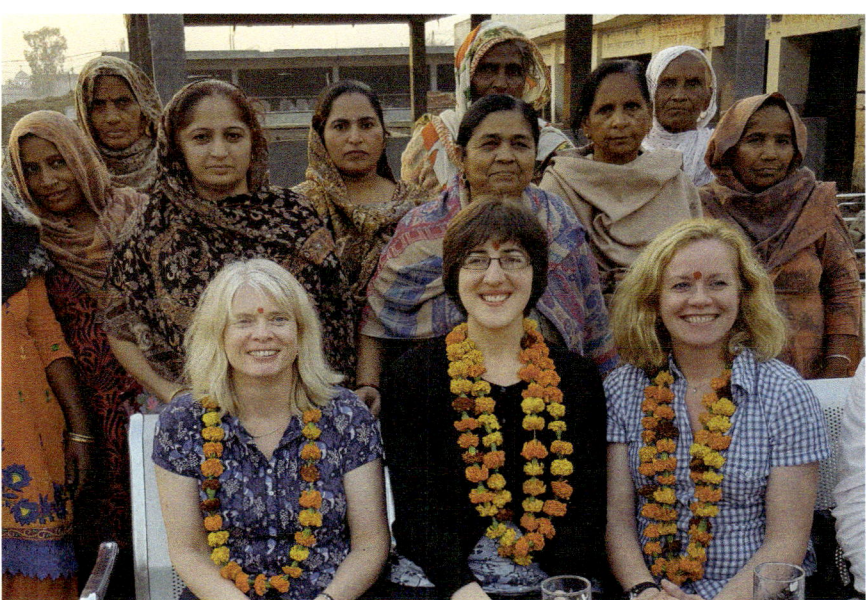

Fig. 5.1. Cathy Dwyer (seated, on the right) and Fritha Langford (seated, middle – with SRUC colleague Marie Haskell, on left) at a gaushala in Karnal, India. Engaging local communities and understanding cultural differences in a non-judgemental manner helps to build relationships to improve animal welfare collaboratively.

(Rayner *et al.*, 2020). In some studies improved knowledge can be associated with changed perceptions (Grigg and Kogan, 2019), which may lead to improved animal welfare. However, other studies suggest that whereas an educational intervention (for children) changed their behaviour in a zoo, the behaviour of the animals, and perhaps their welfare, did not change (Collins *et al.*, 2019).

Education and learning can influence attitudes and beliefs, which play a role in our behaviour towards animals. A Massive Open-access Online Course (MOOC) in animal behaviour and welfare triggered positive attitudinal change in learners across all four areas of attitudinal learning (General Learning, Cognitive Learning, Affective Learning and Behavioural Learning; Watson *et al.*, 2016). Hazel *et al.* (2011) showed that undertaking a course in animal welfare and ethics led to an increase in positive attitudes towards animals classed as 'pests' or 'profit' in veterinary students. In a different approach, the attitudes and beliefs of stockpersons were specifically targeted in a training programme for pig producers, which caused changed stockperson and pig behaviour, relating to improved animal welfare (Hemsworth *et al.*, 1994; Coleman *et al.*, 2000). More generally, education, particularly involving active engagement, can increase empathy (Brunero *et al.*, 2010). Education, therefore, can be targeted at specific groups to improve knowledge and attitudes towards animals, and to raise awareness of specific issues (Fig. 5.2). With education of veterinarians

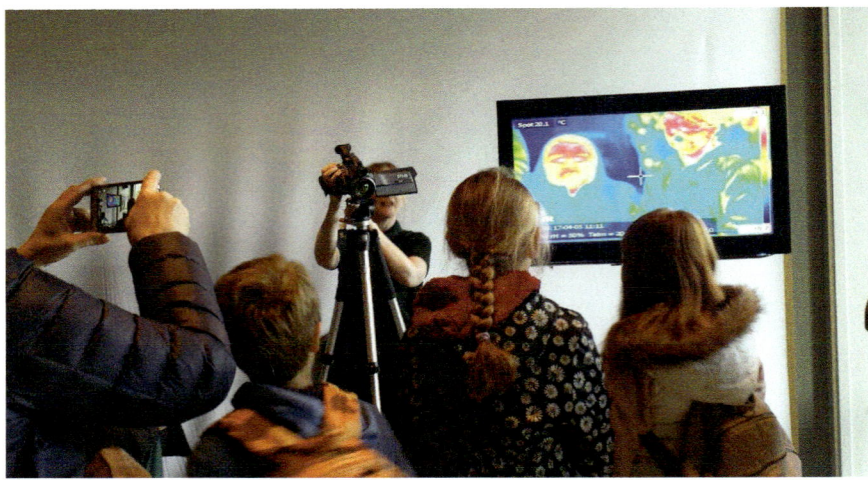

Fig. 5.2. School children at a Science Festival engaging in animal welfare science through the use of thermal imaging to explain heat stress.

Case Study 1: Veterinary Animal Welfare Education Case

In 2011 the Royal (Dick) School of Veterinary Studies at University of Edinburgh founded the Jeanne Marchig International Centre for Animal Welfare Education (the Centre). The Centre aims to improve animal welfare through global veterinary education, recognizing the key role that veterinarians can play as advocates for animal welfare. In 2020 the Royal (Dick) School of Veterinary Studies received the inaugural Animal Welfare Veterinary School of the Year Award from the World Veterinary Association and Ceva.

The Centre approached its mission in a number of ways, considering what should be in a veterinary curriculum, how education was delivered and the impact of other teaching practices, such as the use of live animals as teaching aids. An important component of the work was to address the so-called 'hidden curriculum' where the practical aspects of education and training may inadvertently contradict theoretical teaching. For example, a vet school may adopt comprehensive lecture-based teaching in animal welfare theory, but if students leave those lectures and are then expected to perform aversive experiments or surgical training on live animals, the school is demonstrating that in reality animal welfare is not important, and this is the message that students will absorb. To avoid this, animal welfare theory and practice is themed throughout the curriculum and consideration given to the ethical sourcing and use of animals in teaching and research. Replacing the use of live animals with models, manikins, haptic trainers, computer programs and videos can help to tackle this issue (see Fig. 5.3), and additionally alleviate moral stress and enhance learning among students, as students can practise as often as they wish, without fear of hurting an animal.

Continued

Case Study 1: Continued.

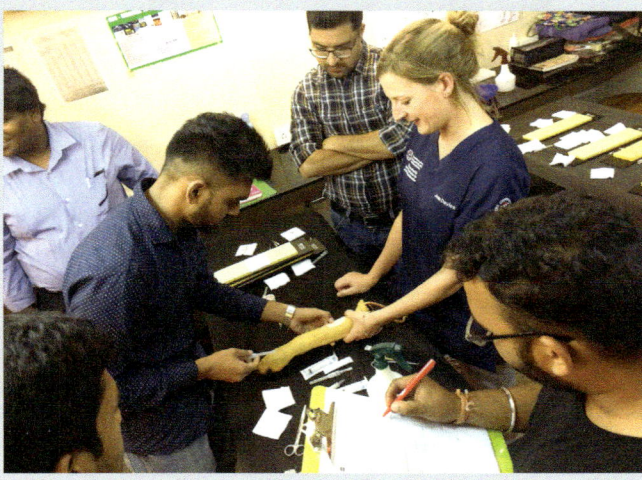

Fig. 5.3. Centre veterinary nurse, Jess Davies, helping students to improve their clinical skills by using a dog's leg model at a clinical skills training workshop in Goa, India. This reduces the need for the use of live animals in veterinary training, and helps to improve student confidence.

In addition thought is given to the sourcing and use of animals for dissection, and to the standards of clinical practice delivered to animals in the vet school. Open discussion of ethically challenging cases and adherence to excellent standards of hospitalization, analgesia and other aspects of clinical care are essential in supporting and demonstrating an institutional commitment to animal welfare. In short, educational establishments have an ethical duty to 'practise what they preach', not just teaching animal welfare theory but reinforcing through their own policies and behaviours that animal welfare is a priority in education. By showing leadership and a commitment to animal welfare at the highest level, we can inspire and educate generations of students who share this same perspective. This holistic and pragmatic approach to animal welfare education has been shared with veterinary schools around the world.

and other professional groups, there is the opportunity for this to be cascaded to clients and animal owners to improve welfare, if these professionals are also taught how to deliver information and to engage with others.

5.3 Animal Welfare Curricula

Although different groups may require different approaches, basic animal welfare knowledge comprises an appreciation of animal sentience and why that matters, and an understanding of welfare needs of animals, and the behavioural and physiological responses of different species when healthy and when unwell. The interdisciplinary nature of animal welfare issues also suggests that an animal welfare education should include legal, societal and ethical aspects, and a range of practical and personal skills.

In addition, there may be specific professional requirements. For veterinarians, there are requirements to meet the 'Day One Competences' (the minimum knowledge, skills and abilities of any newly qualified veterinarian). The World Organisation for Animal Health (OIE) recommendations include a number of competences that are directly related to animal welfare (see Fig. 5.4), such as an ability to assess the welfare status of an animal or group of animals and take corrective action, among other competences indirectly linked to animal welfare (www.oie.int). This requires underpinning knowledge of animal behaviour, physiology and welfare needs, legislation relating to animal welfare and ethical frameworks relating to animal welfare. These skills are focused on ensuring that veterinarians have the knowledge base and skills to safeguard animal welfare. However, to accommodate the changing role of veterinarians in society as educators of clients and the general public, the curriculum

---

Animal welfare means how an animal is coping with the conditions in which it lives. An animal is in a good state of welfare if (as indicated by scientific evidence) it is healthy, comfortable, well nourished, safe, able to express innate behaviour and if it is not suffering from unpleasant states such as pain, fear and distress. Good animal welfare requires disease prevention and veterinary treatment, appropriate shelter (when relevant), management, nutrition, humane handling and humane slaughter/killing. Animal welfare refers to the state of the animal; the treatment that an animal receives is covered by other terms such as animal care, animal husbandry and humane treatment. Veterinarians should be the leading advocates for the welfare of all animals, recognizing the key contribution that animals make to human society through food production, companionship, biomedical research and education.

Specific learning objectives for this competency include the Day One veterinary graduate being able to:

- explain animal welfare and the related responsibilities of owners, handlers, veterinarians and others responsible for the care of animals;
- identify animal welfare problems and participate in corrective actions;
- know where to find up-to-date and reliable information regarding local, national and international animal welfare regulations/standards in order to describe humane methods for:
    - animal production;
    - transport;
    - slaughter for human consumption and killing for disease control purposes.

Fig. 5.4. OIE Day One Competences. (Source: https://www.oie.int/app/uploads/2021/03/dayone-b-ang-vc.pdf, accessed 24 May 2021.)

also needs to expand to encompass skills in discourse, explaining and demonstrating good practice in animal welfare (Dolby and Litster, 2015). There is evidence that veterinarians are also influenced by the perceived 'norms' of their profession, including overlooking behavioural health concerns, or avoiding their educational responsibilities owing to time constraints or a lack of confidence. This can lead to conflict or mismatched expectations between clients and vets (Belshaw *et al.*, 2018; Sumner and von Keyserlink, 2018). Balancing the veterinary curriculum to cover both physical health problems and the behavioural and psychological needs of animals is an essential first step to empowering vets to support clients in delivering better care for pets, equines and livestock. Veterinary students must also have the opportunity to develop communication and debating skills, examine bias and preconceptions, and to explore contentious issues where a diversity of ethical views may make decision making challenging. Veterinarians are often faced with making difficult ethical decisions related to patient care and professional responsibilities. They are expected to advocate on the interests of both human clients and animal patients, even when these interests clash (Batchelor and McKeegan, 2012; Batchelor *et al.*, 2015). Thus, a firm grounding in ethical reasoning, critical thinking and evidence analysis is also an essential component in empowering vets to engage with difficult ethical dilemmas, and advocate for good animal welfare.

Mackay (2020) highlights the potential issue of a 'hidden curriculum' within animal welfare education and the inevitable conflict between the 'objective' and the 'subjective' that is encountered when studying a science with subjective experience at its core. The hidden curriculum is defined as implicit values, beliefs and norms, which are perpetrated by educators who act as behavioural models to the students. Several themes have arisen in relation to the hidden curriculum in medical education, which are especially pertinent to animal welfare education: loss of idealism, emotional socialization and resulting impact on mental health (Cribb and Bignald, 1999). During the process of learning about animal welfare, students may lose their initial idealism in relation to the subject and become more pragmatic and cynical. This enables them to 'survive' the subject matter, but may be problematic if it stifles creativity or causes a loss in self-belief in being able to make a difference. For animal welfare educators, it is therefore important that this is appreciated, and self-reflection of the impact of our own behaviour and practices is maintained.

5.4 Pedagogical Approaches to Teaching Animal Welfare

The essential components of an animal welfare curriculum are fairly widely agreed upon. However, there is a good argument, based on the complex and dynamic nature of animal welfare, to suggest that the teaching of the subject should move away from a traditional lecture-based system towards active learning with a specific focus on problem solving, and acknowledgement of the importance of self-efficacy and communication skills.

Active learning covers a wide range of teaching and learning practices that ask students 'to do something' with course materials, which gives them an experience rather than a purely passive absorption of knowledge. This can be as simple as small-group discussions within a wider lecture format, flipped classrooms where students are given material prior to a classroom session and then spend in-class time applying and investigating this content, through to practicals and visits. Active learning has been used successfully in animal welfare education in various contexts, such as:

- undergraduate animal science students participating in an animal welfare judging contest (Heleski *et al.* 2003);
- scenario use for teaching undergraduate students about welfare assessment (Siegford *et al.*, 2010);
- scenario use in a training course on animal welfare and euthanasia for Indian veterinarians (Rayner *et al.*, 2020);
- small-group discussion and presentations by undergraduate students on an elective animal welfare course (Lord and Walker, 2009);
- interactive videos in an animal behaviour and welfare MOOC (Watson *et al.*, 2016); and
- activity-based events on poultry welfare for high school children (Jamieson *et al.*, 2012).

A particular type of active learning that lends itself to animal welfare education is problem-based learning (PBL). This student-centred teaching method allows students to learn through the experience of working in a small group to discuss and work through how you might solve a particular problem. A key characteristic of PBL is that problems are presented at the beginning of the learning process and are ill-defined (Barrett and Moore, 2010). This means that students are relatively naïve and are starting the process from their own individual levels of knowledge and attitudes towards a problem. PBL tutorials are based on the principles of social constructivism, whereby knowledge is constructed through interaction with others, and education programmes utilizing a PBL approach have been found to be superior to traditional approaches when looking at long-term knowledge retention, acquisition of specific skills and mixed knowledge and skill acquisition (Strobel and van Barneveld, 2009). However group learning also facilitates several other desirable attributes, such as communication skills, teamwork, problem solving, independent responsibility for learning, sharing information and respect for others (Lane, 2008). The use of a specific problem within PBL is thought to increase curiosity in particular subject areas, to ensure that the curriculum is seen as relevant as these problems are seen as real world and pertinent to future professions and to integrate learning across all aspects of the curriculum (Yew and Goh, 2016).

Students on animal welfare programmes generally expect and enjoy practical 'hands-on' teaching involving animals. Clearly, for those students who will require practical skills in their future careers, a level of 'hands-on' learning is necessary in order for them to practise and hone these skills. From the perspective of student wellbeing, some 'hands-on' time with animals has also been found to be beneficial (Wood *et al.*, 2018).There is also good justification for undertaking practicals and visits as it allows full immersion in the sights, sounds and smells of a farm, auction market or abattoir, thus making it possible to contextualize in-class learning. Kolb and Kolb (2017) argue that it is not helpful to separate practical experience outside of the classroom from the within-classroom learning. In order to get the full benefit of this practical experience it is important to integrate action and experience with conceptual analysis and reflection. Therefore, it is not simply the practical 'hands-on' activities that are important but also the classroom-based discussion and both group and individual reflection. It is also very important that educators, as advocates of animal welfare, ensure that any use of animals for 'hands-on' teaching preserves or actually has the potential to improve the welfare of those animals. For instance, stray dogs in shelters may be used to teach surgical neutering skills to veterinary students – this can provide a beneficial opportunity for students to acquire surgical skills, and to control dog populations (Fig. 5.5). However, the training can also be used to teach all facets of dog welfare, beyond just providing an opportunity for developing practical skills. Thus, this provides the students with opportunities for learning how to conduct an ethical analysis of whether neutering is appropriate for the dog, a full clinical examination of each dog, appropriate use of analgesia and anaesthesia with pain assessment, and good hospitalization and post-operative monitoring facilities, which can also benefit the welfare of the dog. This reinforces students' understanding that any teaching using animals is ethically justified and animal-centred.

If possible, students should be actively engaged in the process of ensuring good animal welfare in teaching. They could undertake welfare assessment

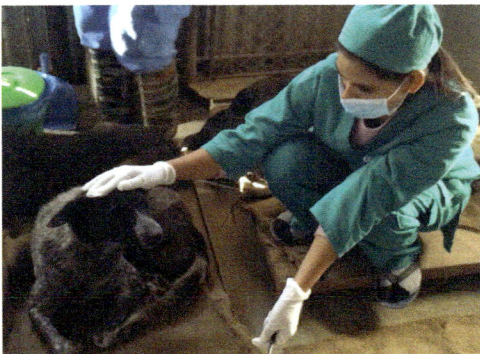

Fig. 5.5. Students engaged in a Capture–Neuter–Return project for stray dogs in Kathmandu, Nepal. In addition to clinical skills, students are exposed to a range of welfare and animal care issues and can be fully engaged in ethical decision making through their participation in the programme.

during teaching activities and be involved with the ethical decision making process on when animals should not be used for particular activities or involved in the design of alternative teaching methods, perhaps using technology that does not involve animals. Mackay (2020) suggests that students could be involved in keeping records on animals used for teaching, which are passed on to each new group, thus ensuring animal welfare is optimized and increasing the sense of community within the student group.

Traditionally education, including animal welfare education, has been delivered in a face-to-face format. However, in recent years there has been a move towards digital education as a tool to deliver animal welfare teaching. For example, the Royal (Dick) School of Veterinary Studies at the University of Edinburgh offers an online MSc in international animal welfare, ethics and law alongside the original on-campus MSc in applied animal behaviour and animal welfare programme. Although online delivery of a subject that appears to require practical application may seem counterintuitive, active learning is still possible in an online environment and there are a number of other benefits to providing education in this format. First, animal welfare is a multidisciplinary subject so digital delivery allows for collaboration across departments, institutions and countries in the production and delivery of content. It also increases accessibility to students who do not have access to an animal welfare programme within their own institution or country, and it may be more affordable to students than an on-campus programme, which may incur travel and living costs as well as international student fees. Finally, digital education generally allows greater flexibility in when students interact with teaching materials, which enables those who are already established in a career to upskill and stay current. This has the potential for significant positive impact on animal welfare as these individuals may already be respected within organizations and industry and potentially have greater influence and reach. Digital education lends itself well to a suite of different active learning technologies including quizzes, synchronous and asynchronous discussions, and video interactions. Learners on an animal welfare MOOC overwhelmingly indicated that the instructor videos were the most impactful instructional strategy (Watson *et al.*, 2016).

In 2020, animal welfare education largely moved to a digital or 'hybrid' format owing to COVID-19. While it is possible to deliver content, engage students in activities and discussion, and undertake assessment in this format, what is most difficult to replace is the sense of community and the learning that takes place during conversation and social interactions outside of the classroom. The presence of an online community reduces feelings of isolation, improves content integration and academic achievement, and increases student satisfaction (Adams and Wilson, 2020). Community is a very important aspect of the learning process and is particularly important if students are undertaking education remotely, but can be achieved through thoughtful use of interactions such as discussion boards, video 'hang-outs' and Q&As.

5.5 Education and Human Behaviour Change

Delivering culturally appropriate education that empowers learners and equips them with both knowledge and skills, and supports inclusivity and action towards improving animal welfare, has been shown to be effective (Fig. 5.6). However, regardless of how comprehensive an animal welfare education curriculum is, or how effective the educational strategies that may be used, animal welfare education may still not translate into human behaviour that supports positive animal welfare. We see this often – for example, vets who do not provide adequate analgesia to their patients (Remnant *et al.*, 2017), or people who choose to engage in detrimental wildlife tourism opportunities when on holiday (Von Essen *et al.*, 2020). The connection between knowledge, attitudes and behaviours is not linear and many other things can impact upon human behaviour – some of which we have already touched upon. Cultural norms can significantly influence behaviour, and be a barrier to change. It may be that international standards of animal welfare do not align with cultural norms and so the person is forced to 'choose'. In such cases culture can be a barrier to delivering good animal welfare (Burton *et al.*, 2012). Similarly, the biggest predictor of future human behaviour is current human behaviour – habit has a very strong influence on what we do and changing habits can be very difficult. So if a pet owner habitually feeds their dog four times each day and

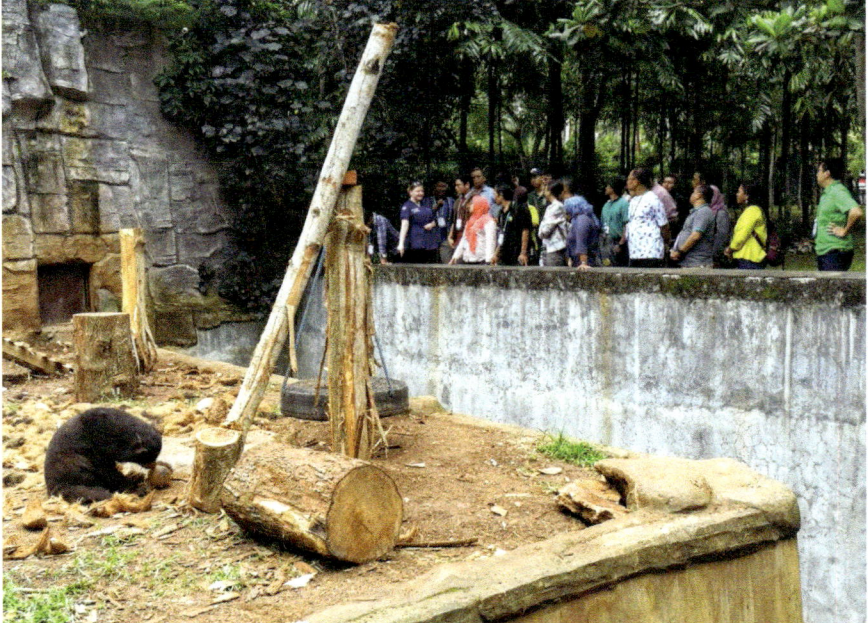

Fig. 5.6. Dr Bacon (standing on left) discussing enrichment opportunities to improve the welfare of rehabilitated bears at a zoo welfare workshop in Lampung, Indonesia.

only exercises them for a few minutes, then even if they are educated about the welfare problems caused by pet obesity, they are likely to find it difficult to change their habits. Other barriers to changing human behaviour also exist as explored elsewhere in this book – see Chapters 2–4. It is for these reasons that effective animal welfare education focuses not only on imparting knowledge but also on developing skills and attitudes, empowering learning to critically evaluate our own behaviour and actions, reflect on past behaviours and develop constructive strategies for modifying behaviour to improve the welfare of animals.

Case Study 2: Effective Postgraduate Education in Animal Welfare

The on-campus MSc in applied animal behaviour and animal welfare at the Royal (Dick) School of Veterinary Studies was the first programme of its type in the world. Initiated by Professor David Wood-Gush in 1990, today it is delivered collaboratively between the University of Edinburgh and SRUC. In the 30 years since the inception of the MSc, over 700 students from all over the world have graduated and have gone on to forge successful careers in research, education, government, veterinary practice, non-governmental and industry organizations (among others). Together they have made significant contributions to the field, resulting in tangible improvements to animal welfare around the world. In 2017, in recognition of this, the MSc, alongside its online sister programme, the MSc in international animal welfare ethics and law (introduced in 2013) won the British Society for Animal Science/Royal Society for the Prevention of Cruelty to Animals (RSPCA) Award for Innovative Developments in Animal Welfare.

There are several reasons why these programmes have been so successful in educating the animal welfare scientists of the future, not least the students themselves and the culture that they bring to the programmes every year. Both the on-campus and online programme attract students from all over the world with very different interests and experiences. Within this melting pot they are given the opportunity to share their experiences and ideas, develop new ideas and interests, and even in some cases question their own beliefs. This is done in an environment where everyone's ideas are seen as important, and therefore should be listened to, but will also be questioned and critically evaluated as part of the learning process.

The collaboration between the University of Edinburgh and SRUC is another notable strength of these programmes, creating one of the largest animal behaviour and welfare research groups in the world. Course leaders on the programmes are research active and leaders in their respective fields so students benefit from this expertise and content is current and relevant. Learning from people who are working in animal welfare and making a 'real' difference is also important as this is inspirational to students and makes a future in animal welfare tangible. Therefore, a number of internationally recognized guest lecturers from research institutions, NGOs and industry also contribute to the programmes. Students thus learn that animal welfare solutions can be implemented in the real world and this can counter the 'loss of idealism' that may affect students on animal welfare programmes.

Continued

Case Study 2: Continued.

An important element of the MSc programme is the dissertation project. This self-directed piece of research brings together the theoretical knowledge and skills developed throughout the programme and allows the student to apply them to an area in which they have a specific interest. Students generate research questions, and work alongside their supervisors to develop a project proposal, submit the project for ethical review and complete all relevant health and safety and risk assessment documentation. This element of project planning is a reality of research and highlights the importance of the 'process' that has to take place prior to research. The students learn a number of technical skills (such as behavioural observation, lab skills, questionnaire development) and personal skills (such as time management and planning, team work and communication, writing and reporting their results). Many of these skills are transferable and beneficial to a number of future careers. The MSc programmes work closely with a number of NGOs, and student projects often involve the analysis and reporting of NGO data, which may otherwise have remained on a database. This provides results that organizations can share with the public or stakeholders, allows evaluation of previous interventions that may promote planning of future activities and, most importantly, this sharing of knowledge with organizations that are working 'at the coal face' has the potential to improve animal welfare in a real and tangible way.

5.6 Conclusions

This chapter has outlined the need for a dynamic, comprehensive and evidence-based approach to developing curricula and pedagogy in animal welfare. It is essential that animal welfare education is holistic, incorporating scientific evidence, ethical reasoning, communication skills and reflective practice. Educators should beware of 'siloing' animal welfare within a discrete lecture series, and should instead aim to ensure that theoretical teaching is enhanced by active PBL, digital resources, and animal interactions that support student engagement in ethical reasoning and animal welfare assessment and improvements. Student interactions with animals in educational settings should be evaluated and ethically justified to ensure that they support good animal welfare practice and reinforce theoretical principles of good animal welfare. Institutional culture should be examined and barriers to delivering good animal welfare in practice addressed, in order to ensure that teaching is not undermined. Delivering effective animal welfare education requires not just interdisciplinary teaching of physiological, behavioural and emotional aspects of welfare, but also interdisciplinary engagement between social and natural sciences to support and empower students to engage and develop skills in moral reasoning, self-reflection and communication.

It is unfortunately common for people working in animal care industries to experience moral stress, burnout and compassion fatigue (Hill *et al.*, 2020). Therefore, within animal welfare education it is important to help students to develop emotional literacy, aid them to express and reflect on challenging emotions, and give them space and support so that they can use these emotions in a constructive way. Reflective practices, such as discussion of the emotional impacts of the exposure to the realities of the use of animals in society, are important components in safeguarding student wellbeing in animal welfare education.

COM-B and Institutional Behaviour: International Collaboration to Deliver Veterinary Nurse Training, Enhanced Veterinary Education and Improved Patient Care

1. Establish capability: Find common ground, build trust

There are many geographic, clinical and cultural differences between vet schools in the UK and Asia, but recognizing commonalities and empathizing with challenges is essential. In many situations, grievous animal welfare problems may be observed in veterinary schools around the world. Understanding why these problems arise (lack of skills, lack of resources, limited drug access, lack of training, habit and cultural norms) is fundamental to addressing them. Insight may be gained through unobtrusive observation, collegiate conversations or more structured discussion and 'needs analysis'. It is essential throughout that personal judgement or ethical discomfort does not impede open and frank communications around what the perceived problems might be, and what the perceived barriers to change are.

2. Motivate: Find a 'hook'

While improving animal welfare might be our focus, it isn't necessarily the priority of a partner institution, so it's important that we analyse what matters to them – is it excellence in veterinary education, developing specialist clinical services, improving their reputation or developing research partnerships? Each of these themes offers an opportunity to engage, and importantly to influence the way animals might be used within veterinary education and research. There may be concerns about the term 'animal welfare' owing to animal rights activism, so by focusing on a 'safer' theme that is of mutual interest we can weave in activities that support good animal welfare without generating concerns.

3. Show opportunities: Model solutions

Once relationships are built, needs and barriers are identified, and a collaborative theme of work established, solutions can be implemented, or if no frame of reference exists, appropriately modelled. An example of this is a project where registered veterinary nurses (RVNs) from the UK worked alongside veterinary clinicians in teaching hospitals in Asia. By modelling the role of the veterinary nurse (a position that does not exist in Asia) we were able to demonstrate their value. This activity enabled vets to see first-hand that properly trained RVNs were not a threat to the role of veterinarians, but actually supported further development of veterinary education, inpatient care and clinical practice standards. As part of this activity, specific infection control protocols, inpatient daily care routines and even a designated cat ward were developed at the hospitals that collaborated.

Continued

Continued.

4. Show opportunities: Demonstrate alternatives

Once on-site activities and enthusiasm were generated, a 'roadmap' for ongoing activities could be developed. For the example of veterinary education, this included visits to our own veterinary hospital from senior management at partnering vet schools. This enabled partners to experience first-hand the different approaches to veterinary education and to clinical hospital management that could potentially be implemented in their own institutions. At the end of this visit, goals were set for replicating some of the activities in the partner institutions. For institutions motivated by research opportunities, demonstrating research methods in animal behaviour through hands-on workshops and discussion facilitated engagement with animal welfare principles.

5. Support new behaviours: Self-efficacy and sustainability

We offer a programme of remote support and mentoring to international colleagues, including developing collaborative Memorandum of Understanding agreements, developing educational resources to provide continuing support to their implementation of agreed activities, and advising and mentoring on pedagogy, curriculum development and research grant development. This holistic combination of practical and philosophical support has always focused very much on empowering the partners to develop their own activities. So far, these include the development of veterinary nursing curricula at three Asian vet schools, investment in clinical facilities for inpatients, development of appropriate clinical and logistical protocols leading to improved hospital management and enhanced student education, and a new Asian research centre in animal welfare.

References

Adams, B. and Wilson, N.S. (2020) Building community in asynchronous online higher education courses through collaborative annotation. *Journal of Educational Technology Systems* 49, 250–261.

Barrett, T. and Moore, S. (2010) *New approaches to Problem-Based Learning*. Routledge, London.

Batchelor, C. and McKeegan, D. (2012) Survey of the frequency and perceived stressfulness of ethical dilemmas encountered in UK veterinary practice. *Veterinary Record* 170, 119.

Batchelor, C., Creed, A. and McKeegan, D. (2015) A preliminary investigation into the moral reasoning abilities of UK veterinarians. *Veterinary Record* 177, 124.

Belshaw, Z., Robinson, N.J., Dean, R.S. and Brennan, M.L. (2018) Owners and veterinary surgeons in the United Kingdom disagree about what should happen during a small animal vaccination consultation. *Veterinary Sciences* 5, 7.

Brunero, S., Lamont, S. and Coates, M. (2010) A review of empathy education in nursing. *Nursing Inquiry* 17, 65–74.

Burton, R.J.F., Peoples, S. and Cooper, M. (2012) Building 'cowshed cultures': A cultural perspective on the promotion of stockmanship and animal welfare on dairy farms. *Journal of Rural Studies* 28, 174–187.

Coleman, G.J. (2010) Educating the public: Information or persuasion? *Journal of Veterinary Medical Education* 37, 74–82.

Coleman, G.J., Hemsworth, P.H., Hay, M. and Cox, M. (2000) Modifying stockperson attitudes and behaviour towards pigs at a large commercial farm. *Applied Animal Behaviour Science* 66, 11–20.

Collins, C., Quirke, T., McKeown, S., Flannery, K., Kennedy, D. and O'Riordan, R. (2019) Zoological education: Can it change behaviour? *Applied Animal Behaviour Science* 220, 104257.

Cribb, A. and Bignold, S. (1999) Towards the reflexive medical school: The hidden curriculum and medical education research. *Studies in Higher Education* 24, 195–209.

De Briyne, N., Vidovic, J., Morton, D.B. and Magalhaes-Sant'Ana, M. (2020) Evolution in the teaching of animal welfare science, ethics and law in European veterinary schools (2012–2019). *Animals* 10, 1238.

Dolby, N. and Litster, A. (2015) Understanding veterinarians as educators: An exploratory study. *Teaching in Higher Education* 20, 272–284.

Fraser, D., Weary, D.M., Pajor, E.A. and Milligan, B.N. (1997) A scientific conception of animal welfare that reflects ethical concerns. *Animal Welfare* 6, 187–205.

Grigg, E.K. and Kogan, L.R. (2019) Owners' attitudes, knowledge and care practices: Exploring implications for domestic cat behaviour and welfare in the home. *Animals* 9, 11.

Hazel, S.J., Signal, T.D. and Taylor, N. (2011) Can teaching veterinary and animal-science students about animal welfare affect their attitude toward animals and human-related empathy? *Journal of Veterinary Medical Education* 38, 74–83.

Heleski, C.R., Zanella, A.J. and Pajor, E.A. (2003) Animal welfare judging teams – A way to interface welfare science with traditional animal science curricula? *Applied Animal Behaviour Science* 81, 279–289.

Hemsworth, P.H., Coleman, G.J. and Barnett, J.L. (1994) Improving the attitude and behaviour of stockpersons towards pigs and the consequences on the behaviour and reproductive performance of commercial pigs. *Applied Animal Behaviour Science* 39, 349–362.

Hill, E.M., LaLonde, C.M. and Reese, L.A. (2020) Compassion fatigue in animal care workers. *Traumatology* 26, 96–108.

Illmann, G., Keeling, L., Melisova, M., Simeckova, M., Ilieski, V. et al. (2014) Mapping farm animal welfare education at university level in Europe. *Animal Welfare* 23, 401–410.

Jamieson, J., Reiss, M., Allen, D., Asher, L., Wathes, C. and Abeyesinghe, S. (2011) Measuring the success of a farm animal welfare education event. *Animal Welfare* 21, 65–75.

Johnstone, E.C.S., Frye, M.A., Lord, L.K., Baysinger, A.K. and Edwards-Callaway, L.N. (2019) Knowledge and opinions of third year veterinary students relevant to animal welfare before and after implementation of a core welfare course. *Frontiers in Veterinary Science* 6, 103.

Kolb, A.Y. and Kolb, D.A. (2017) Experiential learning theory as a guide for experiential educators in higher education. *Experiential Learning & Teaching in Higher Education* 1, Article 7.

Lakestani, N., Aguirre, V. and Orihuela, A. (2015) Farm animal welfare and children: A preliminary study building an attitude scale and evaluating an intervention. *Society & Animals* 23, 363–378.

Lane, E.A. (2008) Problem-based learning in veterinary education. *Journal of Veterinary Medical Education* 35, 631–636.

Lord, L.K. and Walker, J.B. (2009) An approach to teaching animal welfare issues at the Ohio State University. *Journal of Veterinary Medical Education* 36, 276–279.

MacKay, J.R.D. (2020) Discipline-based education research for animal welfare science. *Frontiers in Veterinary Science* 7, 7.

May, S.A. and Silva-Fletcher, A. (2015) Scaffolded active learning: Nine pedagogical principles for building a modern veterinary curriculum. *Journal of Veterinary Medical Education* 42, 332–339.

Rayner, E.L., Airikkala-Otter, I., Bacon, H.J., Walters, H.M., Gamble, L. and Langford, F.M. (2020) Assessment of an educational intervention on the knowledge and attitudes of Indian national veterinarians to animal welfare and euthanasia. *Journal of Veterinary Medical Education* 47, 202–217.

Remnant, J.G., Tremlett, A., Huxley, J.N. and Hudson, C.D. (2017) Clinician attitudes to pain and use of analgesia in cattle: Where are we 10 years on? *Veterinary Record* 181, 400.

Rioja-Lang, F., Bacon, H., Connor, M. and Dwyer, C.M. (2020) Prioritisation of animal welfare issues in the UK using expert consensus. *Veterinary Record* 187, 490.

Siegford, J., Cottee, S. and Widowski, T. (2010) Opportunities for learning about animal welfare from online courses to graduate degrees. *Journal of Veterinary Medical Education* 37, 49–55.

Strobel, J. and van Barneveld, A. (2009) When is PBL most effective? A meta-synthesis of meta-analyses comparing PBL to conventional classrooms. *Interdisciplinary Journal of Problem-Based Learning* 3, 4.

Sumner, C.L. and von Keyserlink, M.A.G. (2018) Canadian dairy cattle veterinarians' perspectives on calf welfare. *Journal of Dairy Science* 101, 10303–10316.

Von Essen, E., Lindsjo, J. and Berg, C. (2020). Instagranimal: Animal welfare and animal ethics challenges of animal-based tourism. *Animals* 10, 1830.

Wood, E., Ohlsen, S., Thompson, J., Hulin, J. and Knowles, L. (2018) The feasibility of brief dog-assisted therapy on university students stress levels: The PAwS study. *Journal of Mental Health* 27, 263–268.

Watson, W.R., Kim, W. and Watson, S.L. (2016) Learning outcomes of a MOOC designed for attitudinal change: A case study of an animal behavior and welfare MOOC. *Computers & Education* 96, 83–93.

Yew, E.H.J. and Goh, K. (2016) Problem-based learning: An overview of its process and impact on learning. *Health Professions Education* 2, 75–79.

6 Moving an Industry: Protecting Farm Animals with Science-based Advocacy

Sara Shields
Humane Society International, Washington, DC, USA

6.1 Introduction

Locked in cages, inside dark, windowless warehouses, the ceaseless suffering of farm animals goes largely unrecognized. It happens in the United States, in China, in Brazil, in South Africa and in every other country where intensive, factory farming has taken hold. But as long as there has been intensive farming, there has been opposition to it. Societal views regarding our responsibilities to animals and our relationships to them are evolving. A shift in sentiment is beginning to usher in change, opening the door for advocacy work around the world.

Farm animal welfare is a programme area for many international animal protection non-governmental organizations (NGOs). While these groups take on a variety of important animal protection issues, the farm animal welfare work stands out for the number of animals affected. In 2019, over 300 million cattle, nearly 1.4 billion pigs and 72 billion chickens (FAO Stat, 2019a) were raised globally for food production. In the United States, in the late 1990s and early 2000s there was a growing recognition of the magnitude of the plight of farm animals and an emphasis on improving tactics and approach. The movement grew and a social justice force that attracted energetic, passionate, dedicated advocates who care deeply and were set on big change began to take hold.

6.2 Work and Life as an Animal Welfare Practitioner

The author (Fig. 6.1) joined the Humane Society of the United States (HSUS) in 2006, and later migrated to Humane Society International (HSI), the expanding international arm. There were not yet many scientists working in farm animal advocacy then, and as an ethologist, it was a niche the author could fill.

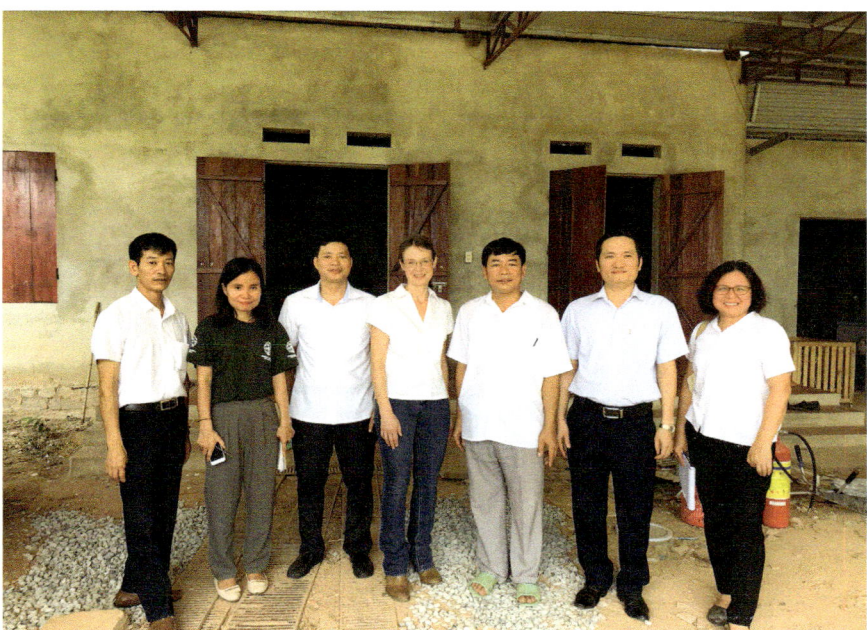

Fig. 6.1. The author (centre) working with Humane Society International colleagues in Vietnam.

The author had finished a degree in animal behaviour from the University of California at Davis, after undergraduate work at Colorado State University and the University of Nebraska. Ethology was largely an underemphasized area in animal science programmes, which were focused on breeding, nutrition and maximizing productivity. A pervasive argument circulated that, if production was good, concerns about welfare were misplaced. Advocates knew there was a firm, science-based counterargument, and that's where ethologists could help. Of course animal welfare science was not new, and the good work of researchers, particularly in Europe, was already available and had begun to permeate US academic institutions, but uptake was slow and there was considerable room to apply the science to advocacy work.

When the author joined, the HSUS Farm Animal Welfare section was responsible for research and analysis. The section developed a collection of white papers exploring each farm animal welfare issue, summarizing the science into comprehensive reports, along with related environmental and public health topics. It was a way to ground advocacy efforts and messaging in science and the addition of new papers to the collection continues to this day.

As the work began to reach new regions of the world, HSI's collaboration with a variety of producers, government offices and institutions associated with agriculture has grown. For the author this means distilling the science into lay terms for different audiences. Whether testifying for a government bill, speaking to a company or showing producers what the science says about managing chickens and pigs for better welfare, the author makes recommendations following the most recent science. The author reviews farm animal welfare standards, audits and certification programmes, and leads HSI's engagement with the International Coalition for Animal Welfare (ICFAW), a group of animal protection organizations officially recognized by the World Organisation for Animal Health (OIE). The author visits farms all over the world, representing every kind of production from cashmere goats in Inner Mongolia to intensive pig farming in Vietnam, and all manner of egg and chicken production throughout Latin America, India and Southeast Asia. It is both wonderful and exhausting but incredibly fulfilling work.

Over the past decade, the number of ethologists working in animal advocacy positions has grown, and there are now trained animal behaviour scientists working with most major animal protection groups. The organizations provide a platform for applying their fervent calling to help animals and their education to real-world animal welfare problems. Ethologists and veterinarians bring credibility to the movement, as well as a critical eye to advocacy efforts, keeping them firmly within the range of scientifically supported facts and analysis. Animal cruelty is an emotive topic, and compassionate people naturally become angry and sad when they are faced every day with animal suffering. While recognizing that the issues are heartbreaking and rightly *should* engender a strong reaction, scientists working in animal advocacy provide objective guideposts, keeping the campaigns steady and accurate, channelling those strong feelings into the most impactful action.

6.3 Improving Animal Welfare as an NGO

There are a plethora of serious, seemingly intractable welfare issues that farm animals endure, including routine painful procedures (such as castration and tail docking, commonly performed without anaesthetic or analgesic interventions), rough or abusive handling, early weaning, long-distance transport, slaughter (sometimes without stunning), physical and metabolic health disorders owing to extremes of genetic selection, and intensive confinement. These problems are common around the world, although the prevalence varies between countries and cultures. While all these issues are important, and organizations care about them all, there has been a strategic focus by HSI on intensive confinement. Ironically, part of the reason for this choice is that it does not take a scientific assessment to see what is wrong – all it takes is a picture and most people recognize the problem. By narrowing efforts to this single issue, organizations are making significant progress.

The problem that occupies most efforts is cage confinement in the egg industry. Battery cages are small wire enclosures, typically confining five to eight egg-laying hens. They are lined in rows and stacked in tiers so that thousands, tens of thousands or even more birds can be housed simultaneously under one roof. In these cages, the hens can barely stretch their wings. They cannot express innate behaviour including perching, foraging, dustbathing or even walking more than a few steps. Most importantly, the restricted space and the barren environment deprive the hens of the opportunity to express nesting behaviour. In motivational analyses, as oviposition (laying eggs) approaches, hens will push more weight for access to a nest box than they will for food (Follensbee, 1993; Cooper and Appleby, 2003). Despite 8000 years of domestication, nesting behaviour is evolutionarily conserved and nest deprivation is a daily frustration for a hen trapped in a battery cage (Fig. 6.2).

The other form of intensive confinement on which organizations focus is gestation crates, the narrow metal stalls used to confine breeding sows. To ease management, conserve space and feed each animal individually, the soon-to-be mother pigs are locked in crates and lined in rows, like parked cars. In a crate, the sow can take a step forwards or backwards, but the stalls are so narrow that she cannot even turn around. She is confined for her entire pregnancy (approximately 114 days) (Fig. 6.3).

While there is little good data on the prevalence of gestation crates around the world, the author has seen them almost everywhere HSI is active. Complicating the issue, it is not just the massive factory farms that utilize these systems; gestation crates and battery cages are used on farms of all sizes. In developing countries, even farms with as few as five pigs use crates, under the misguided belief that the Western system will improve productivity of sows.

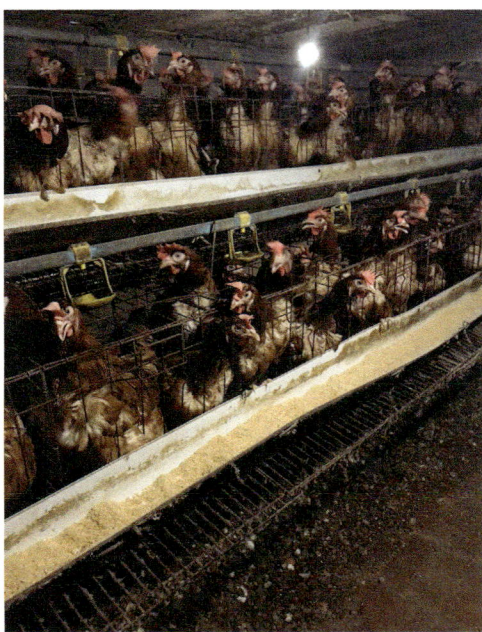

Fig. 6.2. Laying hens in battery cages, Vietnam, 2019.

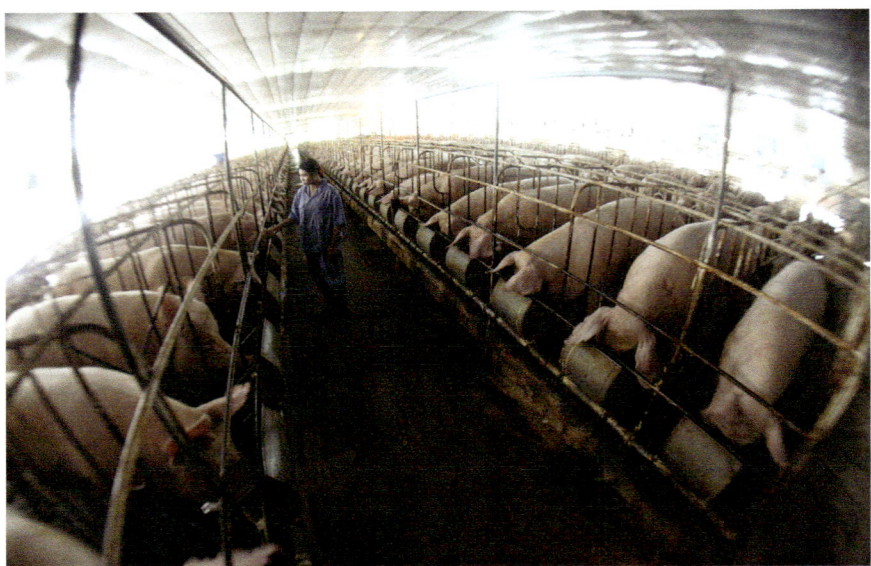

Fig. 6.3. Sows in gestation crates in Vietnam, Xuan Truong.

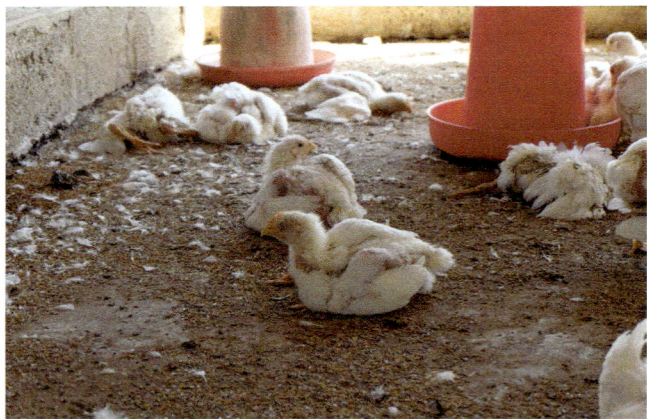

Fig. 6.4. Commercial broiler chickens in India during a drought. Chicken genetic strains from the Western world have exacting environmental and nutritional needs that cannot always be well met, particularly in resource-poor nations.

Smallholders in rural villages often have very few resources and keep the animals to produce food for themselves, perhaps selling a small quantity. There is often a lack of basic information on biosecurity, food safety and animal health, yet, in an attempt to modernize, confinement systems have become entrenched, permeated in agriculture throughout the world.

There is a long history associated with the domination of the factory farming model. The first commercial cages were developed in the United

States in the 1920s and 1930s and from there they spread to Europe (Elson, 2002). By 1970, most egg-laying hens in the developed world were housed in battery cages (Appleby, 2003). Between 1962 and 2012, global egg and pork production increased over 300%. Only broiler chicken meat production grew faster (Windhorst, 2014). 'Agribusiness' emerged from economic incentives to produce more food at lower cost. Operations specialized, intensified and became vertically integrated, owning every stage from feed production to slaughter. The housing systems and 'improved' genetics were exported from the Western world into developing countries (Fig. 6.4). Farms that could not compete were squeezed out, a pattern we see the world over. Consolidation in agriculture is concerning and has been well covered by many authors (e.g. Pollan, 2006; Imhoff, 2010).

While animal welfare is still a relatively new concept in many developing regions, it is slowly taking hold. In some regions basic concepts are needed, including even just understanding the term, 'animal welfare'. In other regions animal welfare is quite advanced and taken without question. There is a pervasive view, even a prejudice, that developed countries have better welfare, which is true in some cases (effective stunning of cattle before slaughter, for example); however, it is not always the case that welfare is worse in the developing world. For example, smallholdings or shepherd-tended herds in Africa, Asia and Latin America generally permit the expression of most natural behaviour. Also, in some communist countries, where agriculture is a social priority, this has implications for farm animals. In these cases, veterinary care is free and overseen by a trusted, accessible veterinarian in a local office. In contrast, the current shortage of large animal veterinarians leaves small farmers in the United States with few and expensive options, forcing them to perform their own animal health interventions. Large industrial poultry producers have too many animals to provide individualized veterinary care. Whistleblowers and investigators have come to HSUS documenting hundreds of sick or injured birds on massive poultry farms.

While there is growing support for higher-welfare systems, there remains a stubborn opposition. This opposition seems to be perpetuated by the international industry, which is slow to change. After speaking at events in Chile, China and Vietnam over the past 5 years, the author noticed that the debate in these regions over battery cages is about 10 years behind the United States and about 20 years behind the European Union. Older studies detailing the challenges of cage-free egg production continue to fuel debate.

6.4 Overcoming Challenges

Farm animal welfare is an intractable problem. Growing animals for food production is deeply embedded in the culture and history of most human societies, and the demand for animal protein has been on a steep, upwards trajectory for as long as records have been kept. As countries become more affluent, their populations tend to increase consumption of animal products, setting the stage for the growth of industrial farms and a steady increase in the number of crated and caged animals. Factors driving this dietary shift in urban societies include precooked convenience foods and mass marketing (Milford *et al.*, 2019), along with social-psychological factors such as perceived symbolic links between meat eating and status (Chan and Zlatevska, 2019).

Furthering the meat consumption trend, the suffering of animals is largely outside of the public's purview, out of mind for the typical consumer, who prefers not to know how the animals were raised and slaughtered (Rothgerber, 2020). Even as people love their pets, many dismiss farm animals with a nervous laugh. In the early efforts of the US farm animal welfare movement, activists tried to confront the cognitive disconnect with graphic imagery comparing the consumption of farm animals to the eating of cats and dogs. This was not met with the response hoped, consistent with the scholarly works demonstrating that direct confrontation is not usually effective to change human behaviour (Ahluwalia, 2000; Goldberg *et al.*, 2020), as discussed in Chapters 2–4 of this book. Oblivious to the environmental and social externalities, consumers continue to make purchasing decisions based on taste, convenience and price. The ready availability of inexpensive animal products creates an expectation among consumers that food businesses are eager to fill.

The most effective way to address the issue was a long-deliberated topic in the farm animal protection movement, and many bright minds have contributed thoughtful analysis. While the discussion continues, a good working model has emerged and is collectively employed by many international farm animal protection groups. A combination of policy and corporate outreach backed by science is driving steady, gradual progress around the world.

The obvious place to begin protecting animals is with legislative change, which is where the early movement directed its initial efforts. Following the 1964 publication *Animal Machines* (Harrison, 1964), a burgeoning farm animal protection effort began in England. Policy makers, seeking fact-based information on which to base legislative decisions, turned to scientists for guidance, and the field of farm animal welfare science emerged. The public's intuitive reaction to intensive confinement systems was tested in the animal behaviour laboratory.

In 1989, Marian Dawkins and Sylvia Hardie measured the space occupied by hens performing normal movements, finding that white hens occupied a mean area of 475 cm^2 while standing and 540–1006 cm^2 while turning around (Dawkins and Hardie, 1989). The legal minimum for cage space in a 1986 EU Directive required only 450 cm^2 (Council Directive 86/113/EEC, 1986). This simple, yet powerful demonstration that the space afforded hens in cages was far too small remains a key paper and was used as part of the legal arguments in India that cages should be banned (Case Study 1). The search for a commercially viable alternative to the battery cage helped propel legislative progress. The 1988 Swedish Animal Welfare Act had already mandated a switch from conventional battery cages to alternative housing systems (Fossum *et al.*, 2009) and Switzerland banned battery cages in 1992 (Appleby, 2003). A ban on battery cages throughout the EU was finally passed in 1999 and took full effect in 2012. The International Egg Commission was strongly opposed (Appleby, 2003).

> **Case Study 1: Farm Animal Protection Laws in the United States and India**
>
> In the United States, the first law prohibiting the confinement of gestating sows passed in Florida in 2002. The political influence of US agribusiness prevented any sweeping federal laws, and the only real path for protecting animals on the farm was state-level ballot initiatives, where voters could weigh in directly. While legislators are often beholden to agricultural industries, voters will almost always pass measures preventing animal cruelty. After the success in Florida, ballot initiatives followed in Arizona in 2006 and California in 2008, both efforts led by the HSUS and a coalition of national and local animal protection groups. These historic successes built momentum and in a welcome move, legislatures in Colorado and Oregon passed laws phasing out sow stalls. As of this writing there are now eight US states with cage-free laws and ten prohibiting or phasing out the use of gestation crates.
>
> Following legislative progress in Europe and the United States, one of the other most important successes has been in India, where contrasting forces shape the movement in striking ways. India is the world's second most populous nation and is expected to overtake China in 2027 (United Nations, 2019). While India is one of the fastest-growing egg-producing countries worldwide (the number of laying hens tripled between 1996 and 2016, with egg production growing by almost 300%; Windhorst, 2019), it also struggles with poverty and human malnutrition (Singh, 2020). In other countries with substantial poverty, animal welfare can be a difficult discussion, as policy makers are often uninterested, given the humanitarian crises they are facing. However, India's culture of deference towards animals, rooted in Hinduism, reduces the resistance. The people of India 'get it' when you talk about animal welfare, opening the door for potential progress.
>
> The Indian Prevention of Cruelty to Animals (PCA) Act was enacted in 1960. Section 11(1)(e) of the Act specifically forbids the keeping or confinement of 'any animal in any cage or other receptacle which does not measure sufficiently in height, length and breadth to permit the animal a reasonable opportunity for movement'. In 2012, the Animal Welfare Board, a statutory body of the Government of India, determined that battery cages contravened the PCA Act and 26 of 29 Indian states supported this interpretation. The matter was taken up by the courts and in 2018 the High Court of Delhi issued an interim order prohibiting the construction of new battery cage facilities, which remains in effect as of this writing.

While laws aimed at protecting animals are important and necessary, true progress for farm animals has been advanced by approaching the problem from multiple angles. For any animal welfare issue, a thorough examination of the leverage points, the main influencers that are supporting the problematic practices, is key to change. The underlying driver of inhumane conditions on the farm is price pressure to produce mass quantities of uniform product at a low cost. In animal agriculture, this is primarily the result of competition between suppliers to offer the lowest cost to the grocery, food service, restaurant and hospitality companies that comprise the market for animal products.

For this reason, the farm animal protection movement focuses on big corporations, the companies exerting these price pressures and unknowingly causing the animals to suffer through their buying decisions. Major brands have both the power to change food production, while also being sensitive to brand image, which makes them good campaign targets.

In the early 2000s, the HSUS started a vigorous corporate outreach campaign, meeting with companies across the nation (Shields et al., 2017). The author often participated as the scientific voice at many of these meetings. At first, HSUS was usually passed to company public relations and legal departments and because there was little animal welfare understanding as well as a lack of trust, HSUS's concerns were largely dismissed. However, over approximately the last decade, there has been a growing awareness of labour, environmental and animal welfare issues, and the roles of multinational companies in perpetuating these problems. Companies are culpable for the conditions that emerge in their supply chains. With the growing realization that their purchasing decisions impact people, animals and the environment, corporate social responsibility (CSR) programmes gained more traction, with whole departments dedicated to addressing social issues.

The public sometimes doubts the true motivation of these companies – are they really concerned or just trying to appease their customers? The animal protection movement decided it did not really matter, whether for selfish or altruistic reasons, the results for the animals could be the same. When large companies, with expansive, international supply chains decide to do the right thing, it can literally change the world. This changing CSR landscape opened the door for advocates, and now companies come to us for assistance and many fruitful partnerships have emerged.

HSI now works with companies around the world to make public-facing commitments to rid their supply chains of cages and crates. Many multinational companies are headquartered in Europe or the United States, from where they can promulgate policies affecting farm animals in distant geographies, in places where animal welfare is just beginning to take root. Well-recognized brand names can influence society. Well-placed messaging improves public understanding and acceptance, mainstreaming animal welfare and changing the trajectory of consumer sentiment.

6.4.1 Implementing commitments

While well over 200 major brands have public-facing cage- and crate-free policies, enacting those policies can be logistically challenging in regions of the world where the supply of cage-free eggs and crate-free pork is limited.

Companies sometimes do not act on their promises, especially if there is staff turnover or if finding a good supply proves difficult. Following on the success of the US and European campaigns, many animal protection groups are expanding their efforts into new countries. In Asia, the location of approximately half of the world's pigs (FAO Stat, 2019b) and chickens (FAO Stat, 2019c), cage-free production is just starting to take hold and there is increasing focus and attention on this region.

Changing the Behaviour of Companies and Producers

Implementation is best achieved with support, for both companies (buyers) and producers (sellers). To assist, HSI brings technical knowledge directly to egg farmers by holding workshops, webinars, presentations, farm tours and other events. HSI connects farmers with experts from all over the world. One of the obstacles to producing eggs in an alternative housing system is that cage-free production requires a greater level of skill and husbandry than battery cages. Keeping large flocks of cage-free hens together without high levels of mortality, feather pecking and keel bone fractures requires study and experience. HSI brings researchers, written materials and successful cage-free producers with well-established aviary and barn production systems to new regions. HSI gives high-welfare farmers a platform to talk about their success. Genetics companies, housing equipment manufacturers and certifiers provide a wealth of information and we facilitate dissemination of their technical knowledge and experience. Egg producers are interested not only for the growing market, but because many of them simply feel it is the right thing to do. Initial resistance is often replaced by pride in their higher-welfare systems.

Case Study 2: Reducing Poverty and Improving Animal Welfare Through Direct Marketing

Companies may combine their animal welfare policies with other CSR goals, placing them into an overarching sustainability framework. Some good examples are emerging where human, environmental and animal welfare goals are part of a company's core identity. Toks, a company operating 84 restaurants under several brand names in 20 cities throughout Mexico, serves over 21 million consumers per year. One of their business fundamentals is that 'there is no successful company in a failed society'. Addressing poverty is integral to their business model. They do this with projects working with poor rural communities by incorporating small business enterprises directly into their restaurant supply chains. They have projects for coffee, jams, granola and spices, which are purchased from usually women-owned enterprises, incorporating these products into their menus. Working with HSI in 2016, Toks became the first Mexican restaurant company to commit to a cage-free egg and crate-free pork supply chain. They are proud to help both people and animals together and smartly capitalize on the good work they are doing in their marketing communications. Customers are loyal because they are supporting good causes. It is a win–win–win–win model for the animals, rural farmers, Toks and consumers alike.

Direct marketing works in other regions of the world as well, such as in Africa and India. Happy Hens, a cooperative of small egg farmers that supply major grocery and hospitality outlets in India, has grown from a single farm to over 20 in 2020 and they now sell to over 100 stores in 5 cities. By supporting smallholders in direct marketing of cage-free eggs to upscale, urban businesses, they address both food security and animal welfare. In India, South Africa and Chile, networks of small farmers are beginning to organize, and are poised to be a balancing voice to the industrial producers in trade organizations, which often speak for the whole egg industry.

6.4.2 Global progress

The dual approach with both legislative and corporate policy change, along with animal welfare standards and certification schemes, has ushered in major advances and there is now a snowballing global movement away from battery cages and gestation crates. When the HSUS cage-free campaign started in 2005, the proportion of hens in alternative, cage-free systems was less than 4% in the United States (Shields *et al.*, 2017). Over approximately the next decade, the entire industry began to transform. The number of cage-free hens began to grow exponentially, reaching 15% in 2017 and 20%

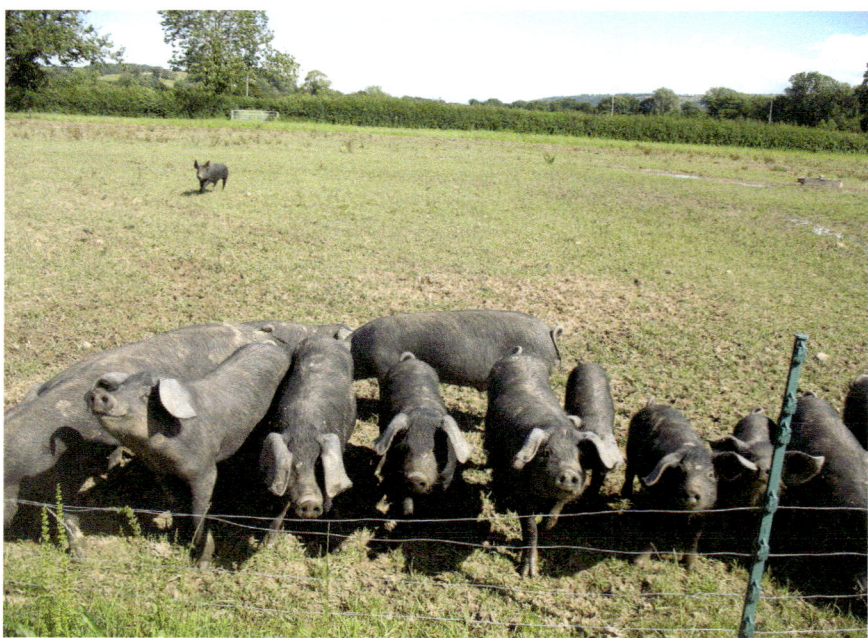

Fig. 6.5. Organically reared pigs in Bristol, England.

in 2019. By May 2021, the number of hens raised in cage-free systems was over 30% of the total US hen population (US Department of Agriculture, 2021). Egg production in both the EU (EC, 2020) and Australia (Australian Eggs Limited, 2019) is now about half cage-free. In 2018 the OIE passed a new chapter in its *Terrestrial Animal Health Code* favouring group housing for sows.

Every company policy announcement, international standard and legislative advance is a victory, and we celebrate these regularly. However, the farm animal protection movement focuses on where we want to be in 20 years, and this guides much of the global effort. Of course, animal protection groups want the animals out of cages yesterday, but organizations are pragmatic and understand that moving an entire global industry takes time. Strong economic forces, societal expectations and the entrenched history must be overcome. The number of animals in cages and crates rises naturally with human population growth. HSI aims to change this trajectory, to flatten the line in the midterm, with the ultimate goal of ending confinement systems forever. Animal protection groups are patient but unyielding, always on the lookout for new science and innovation that will help improve the lives of farm animals and free them faster.

6.5 Conclusions

Every single day, millions of animals languish in confinement systems. There is an urgent need for action, and farm animal advocates need help to be successful. There is a role for everyone, from artists designing fliers to technology experts creating websites, to everyday consumers making careful purchasing decisions in the grocery aisle. Animal welfare practitioners are particularly well positioned to make an impact.

What ethologists/academics can do:

- Study the solutions, not just the problems. Do not hold back progress by sowing doubt. Finding the challenges in cage- and crate-free systems is easy, and these are already well established. The movement needs the brilliant minds in academia to find the answers and help overcome the challenges. The status quo is unacceptable, and we must do better.
- Don't be too neutral. Being objective is an important tenet of science, so studies often stop short of drawing strong conclusions. However, this creates a situation that industry seizes on to deny the problems.
- Be vocal in your convictions that we must do better for the animals. University affiliates are particularly strong voices that can sway the debate. Too often the heavy lifting is left to the NGOs because academics are timid. The welfare of animals is too important. Be the voice the animals need and do not ask for too little.

What governments can do:

- Subsidize the transition to higher-welfare farms. Provide tax breaks to producers who are willing to invest in cage/crate-free systems.
- Stop incentivizing factory farming with subsidies on inputs such as feed.
- Introduce legislation to protect animals on the farm, during transport and at slaughter.
- Offer training and assistance to producers exploring cage- and crate-free housing systems.

What farmers can do:

- Continue to innovate. By working directly with the animals every day, farmers are best positioned to forge new ground. Keep being the pioneers of new, higher-welfare systems.
- Accept change gracefully. No business is static, and only those that can grow and adapt to evolving consumer sentiment and scientific and technological advances will thrive. Be aware of status quo bias, the tendency to overvalue what is, and undervalue other potential options.
- Set the example. There is good reason to tout higher-welfare systems. Communicate your choice to your peers and demonstrate how it can be done.

What food businesses can do:

- Enact public-facing animal welfare policies and implement them. Commit to purchasing only 100% cage/crate-free animal products within an ambitious timeline.
- Make it easy for consumers. With so many important issues to contend with, food choices can be overwhelming. Offer easy, high-welfare alternatives with clear, simple labelling.
- Communicate your purchasing policies to the public. Use animal welfare as a marketing tool by explaining your purchasing policies and the value of animal welfare.
- Offer more non-animal alternatives. Join the plant-based movement and substitute animal products with healthy and delicious vegan options.

What everyone can do:

- Vote with your food spending. One of the most important actions that people can take is to make conscientious food choices. Every food purchase is a vote for or against the welfare of farm animals.
- Get involved. Volunteer, write letters, share your experiences on social media. Be a part of the growing public support for farm animal welfare.
- Support farmers and companies doing right by the animals. Ask grocery stores to carry cage-free eggs or plant-based alternatives.
- Set an example for others. Sometimes the most effective way to change others is simply by demonstrating that compassionate food choices are easy and delicious. The Meatless Mondays campaign is a way to frame the discussion in a positive light, promoting gradual change.

While the suffering of farm animals is immense in scope and scale, there is so much reason to be hopeful. Major victories come regularly and the movement thrives on that success. Animal protection groups are emboldened by the changes. Compassion is a universal value, shared by people the world over. It is definitely not the case that people don't care about farm animals; they usually just don't know. This movement is a natural progression of expanding moral and scientific understanding. There is no better time to become a part of the humane world.

6.6 Recommended Resources

- Humane Society International, www.hsi.org (accessed 2 April 2021).
- Farm Animals Responsible Minimum Standards Initiative, www.farms-initiative.com (accessed 2 April 2021).
- World Organisation for Animal Health, www.oie.int/en (accessed 2 April 2021).

Acknowledgements

The author is grateful to her colleagues across the world, whose dedication, perseverance, talent, intelligence and endless compassion save animals every day. The author is also grateful to her mentors and teachers along the way, whose patience and support have helped the author become a better advocate.

References

Ahluwalia, R. (2000) Examination of psychological processes underlying resistance to persuasion. *The Journal of Consumer Research* 27(2), 217–232.

Appleby, M.C. (2003) The European Union ban on conventional cages for laying hens: History and prospects. *Journal of Applied Animal Welfare Science* 6(2), 103–121.

Australian Eggs Limited (2019) Australian Eggs Limited annual report. Available at: www.australianeggs.org.au/who-we-are/annual-reports (accessed 21 November 2020).

Chan, E.Y. and Zlatevska, N. (2019) Jerkies, tacos, and burgers: Subjective socioeconomic status and meat preference. *Appetite* 132, 257–266.

Cooper, J.J. and Appleby, M.C. (2003) The value of environmental resources to domestic hens: A comparison of the work-rate for food and for nests as a function of time. *Animal Welfare* 12(1), 39–52.

Council Directive 86/113/EEC (1986) Laying down minimum standards for the protection of laying hens kept in battery cages. EEC, Brussels.

Dawkins, M. and Hardie, S. (1989) Space needs of laying hens. *British Poultry Science* 30(2), 413–416.

EC (2020) EU market situation for eggs: Committee for the Common Organisation of the Agricultural Markets. Available at: http://www.avicola-forli.com/userfiles/file/Uova_UE_rapporto.pdf (accessed 2 April 2021).

Elson, A. (2002) Half a century of egg production – The industry's development from 1962 to 2012. *Poultry International* 41(5), 8–17.

FAO Stat (2019a) 72,118,780,000 chickens; 324,520,000 cattle and 1,316,770,000 pigs were slaughtered. Available at: www.fao.org/faostat/en/#data (accessed 6 February 2021).

FAO Stat (2019b) 430,401,827 pigs in Asia and 850,320,154 globally in 2019 Available at: www.fao.org/faostat/en/#data (accessed 6 February 2020).

FAO Stat (2019c) 15,839,266,000 chickens in Asia and 25,915,318,000 globally in 2019 Available at: www.fao.org/faostat/en/#data (accessed 6 February 2020).

Follensbee, M.E., Duncan, I.J.H. and Widowski, T.M. (1993) Quantifying the nesting motivation of domestic hens. *Journal of Animal Science* 70(Suppl. 1), 164.

Fossum, O., Jansson, D.S., Etterlin, P.E. and Vågsholm, I. (2009) Causes of mortality in laying hens in different housing systems in 2001 to 2004. *Acta Veterinaria Scandinavica* 51, 3.

Freire, R., Appleby, M.C. and Hughes, B.O. (1996) Effects of nest quality and other cues for exploration on pre-laying behaviour. *Applied Animal Behaviour Science* 48(1), 37–46.

Goldberg, M.H., Carmichael, C.L. and Hardin, C.D. (2020) Counter-argument self-efficacy predicts choice of belief-defense strategies. *European Journal of Social Psychology* 50(2), 438–447.

Harrison, R. (1964) *Animal Machines*. Vincent Stuart Publishers Ltd., London.

Imhoff, D. (2010) *The CAFO Reader: The Tragedy of Industrial Animal Factories*. University of California Press, Berkeley, California.

Milford, A.B., Le Mouël, C., Bodirsky, B.L. and Rolinski, S. (2019) Drivers of meat consumption. *Appetite* 141, 104313.

Pollan, M. (2006) *The Omnivore's Dilemma: A Natural History of Four Meals*. Bloomsbury, London.

Rothgerber, H. (2020) Meat-related cognitive dissonance: A conceptual framework for understanding how meat eaters reduce negative arousal from eating animals. *Appetite* 146, 104511.

Shields, S., Shapiro, P. and Rowan, A. (2017) A decade of progress toward ending the intensive confinement of farm animals in the United States. *Animals* 7(5), 40.

Singh, A. (2020) Childhood malnutrition in India. In: Bhattacharya, S. (ed.) *Perspective of Recent Advances in Acute Diarrhea*. Intech Open, London, pp. 1–25.

Windhorst, H.-W. (2014) Global egg production dynamics – Past, present and future of a remarkable success story. International Egg Commission. Special economic report.

Windhorst, H.-W. (2019) Patterns and dynamics of the egg industry in India. *Zootecnica International*, April. The International Egg Commission, London. Available at: https://zootecnicainternational.com/featured/patterns-dynamics-egg-industry-india/ (accessed 22 April 2021).

United Nations (2019) World population prospects: Highlights. United Nations. Available at: https://population.un.org/wpp/Publications/Files/WPP2019_Highlights.pdf (accessed 21 November 2020).

US Department of Agriculture (2021) Egg markets overview. US Department of Agriculture, Agricultural Marketing Service, 28 May. Available at: https://www.ams.usda.gov/sites/default/files/media/Egg%20Markets%20Overview.pdf?&~nfopt(file-Distorted=94413 (accessed 31 May 2021).

7 Applying the Science of Animal Welfare to Build More Responsible Food Supply Chains: Reflections from a Corporate Sustainability Professional

Priya Motupalli
IKEA Food, Malmö, Sweden

7.1 Introduction

7.1.1 Welcome to IKEA Food

IKEA Food is a multinational food business under the larger IKEA home furnishing brand. Animal products feature as a component of the larger food offer, with iconic products like the Swedish meatball (containing pork, beef and eggs) being among the most popular products globally, with 1 billion sold annually.

Originally, the food business was seen purely as a way to help IKEA sell more furniture, as its founder, Ingvar Kamprad found it 'hard to do business with customers on an empty stomach'. The 2013 horsemeat scandal – wherein traces of equine DNA were discovered in frozen IKEA meatballs in Europe – changed this approach. The backlash both damaged IKEA's reputation and led to financial consequences. This incident highlighted the potential risk that the food business could be to the brand, but it also lent impetus to the idea that food could play a significant role in delivering on IKEA's vision 'to create a better everyday life for the many people'.

7.1.2 Development of an animal welfare strategy

In large part, the IKEA Food business hopes to deliver on the IKEA vision through their People and Planet Positive Strategy (PPP), which describes the sustainability ambitions across the IKEA value chain. Supporting more sustainable animal agriculture (MSAA), including better animal welfare, is a key way for the food business to contribute to this strategy. Animal welfare is intentionally positioned as an integrated part of our MSAA ambitions such that, at least for IKEA Food, an animal agricultural system cannot be considered 'responsible' if it does not provide a decent quality of life for animals.

The application of animal welfare science frameworks was essential in determining what a decent quality of life looks like for individual species in the food supply chain. The author used the conceptual framework developed by Fraser *et al.* (1997; see Chapter 3) to focus on animals' physical and mental health and to ensure that animals have opportunities to express important natural behaviours. This framework also highlights that in addition to being a science-based concept, animal welfare is also a value-based one.

As a customer-driven company, IKEA Food recognized that the natural living component of animal welfare and opportunity for positive experiences would align most closely with our customers' and internal co-worker values as they relate to animal welfare. As discussed in Chapter 3, these aspects of animal welfare are generally the biggest gap between what a customer *believes* is happening within food supply chains and what is *actually* happening (Ventura *et al.*, 2016; Rault *et al.*, 2020), as the focus has traditionally been, and for the most part continues to be, on the physical health component of animal welfare. While the requirements *also* focus on physical health, IKEA Food wanted its vision for MSAA to close this gap where possible, allowing animals to have some level of agency and being mindful of *wants* in addition to *needs*.

When considering direct implementation (i.e. actual species-specific requirements) we looked to the Five Domains Model (Mellor, 2017), as described in Chapter 1, as well as to the existing body of research and practice related to animal pain, space allowances, enrichment, environmental conditions, behavioural needs and welfare outcome measures. These data and information came from three main avenues: scientific journals (e.g. *Applied Animal Behaviour Science, Applied Animal Welfare Science, Animal Welfare, Frontiers in Veterinary Science* etc.); regular discussions with a network of academics, students, consultants and other sustainability professionals; and through attending conferences with an applied focus, such as the International Society for Applied Ethology annual conference. In addition, we also sought feedback from suppliers and non-governmental organizations (NGOs), worked in partnership with agricultural consultants (FAI Farms) and benchmarked the requirements against existing legislation and certifications.

This approach was helpful especially where the science lacked consensus, clarity or had gaps. In this way IKEA Food favoured progress over perfection – moving towards developing a strategy that had the potential to provide animals with a decent quality of life even when the way forward had not yet been directly prescribed in the literature. As this way of working comes with a level of uncertainty, it naturally fosters a healthy level of pushback – but the alternative, maintaining the status quo, was not in line with the business's entrepreneurial mindset. IKEA Food also tapped into its employees' values by conducting a cross-functional co-worker survey asking them to rank the various sustainability topics proposed as part of the broader development of IKEA Food's contribution to PPP – animal welfare came out as both a key risk and a key opportunity for three of the major regions IKEA operates in (North America, Asia Pacific and Europe), highlighting an internal drive to move forward on this topic.

Integration of the scientific frameworks, published research and multi-stakeholder input resulted in what is called the Better Programmes (BPs). These species-specific programmes frame the IKEA Food vision for MSAA at the farm level by focusing on three key areas: animal welfare, environmental management and public health. Rather than focusing on a singular issue or commitment it was important for IKEA Food to think about the *systems* they wanted to stand behind and promote. This strategy, thinking about the system as a whole and the interconnections between humans, animals and the environment, has become even more urgent during the COVID-19 pandemic. In response to the pandemic, the United Nations Environment Programme (UNEP) identified deforestation and land-use change, intensive animal agriculture and antimicrobial resistance among the key drivers for zoonosis transmission (UNEP, 2020). All these drivers are addressed in some way with the BPs approach.

Case Study 1: Finding the Connections

Amidst COVID-19, several global businesses have pledged to 'build back better', referring to economic recovery policies that strengthen commitments for emissions reductions, reversing biodiversity loss, increasing circularity in supply chains and promoting behaviour change. These focus areas are deemed essential to building a resilient global economy that can withstand future system shocks and reduce the likelihood of their occurrence (OECD, 2020). To date, animal welfare has largely been absent from the conversation. The continued successful integration and prioritization of animal welfare as a business issue will rely on the ability of researchers, sustainability professionals, NGOs and the interested public to tap into the interconnectedness of animal welfare with human and environmental well-being. We need to collectively ask: *how can animal welfare be part of the solution?*

Emerging evidence suggests a link between improved animal welfare and improved immune function. Environments that are more complex, offer animals more choices and allow animals to behave naturally through the provision of enrichment (Fig. 7.1) can fundamentally alter their ability to withstand a disease challenge (van Dixhoorn *et al.*, 2016; Brown *et al.*, 2018; Tatemoto *et al.*, 2019).

As the understanding of this link improves, it has been postulated that a focus on animal welfare has the potential to be a type of 'preventative medicine' (Dawkins, 2019). This focus offers us an opportunity to reduce antibiotics usage – the overuse and misuse of antibiotics, including in animal farming, is connected to the major public health challenge of antimicrobial resistance (O'Neill, 2015). It also contributes to a more resilient model of animal farming that is less susceptible to the

Continued

Case Study 1: Continued.

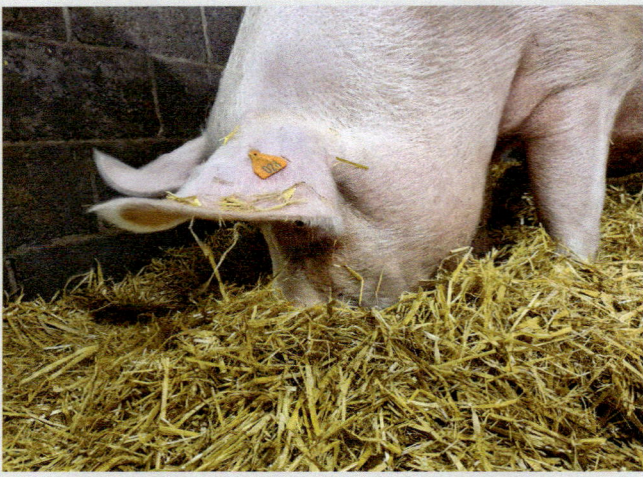

Fig. 7.1. Sow expressing natural rooting behaviour via the provision of straw. (© M. Farish, SRUC.)

devastating impact of recent epidemics like the African swine fever (ASF) outbreak in 2018.

While severe production and animal losses in Asia have been the most obvious impact (OIE, 2020) of ASF, the disruption in the Chinese pork industry led to an increased demand for alternatives to pork. In an effort to meet this global demand, Brazil increased their chicken and beef production reportedly by continuing to clear parts of the Amazon rainforest (Bradsher and Tang, 2019). Deforestation for agricultural purposes has long been recognized as a significant contributor to climate change (IPCC, 2019).

While these links are complex and imperfect, the author argues that considering animal welfare, particularly a renewed focus on providing for opportunities to express natural behaviour, will only support businesses in their quest to 'build back better', as this will have knock-on effects connected to human and environmental well-being by creating a more robust and resilient system. This is still an emerging area, but a promising one for application and quantification in food supply chains.

In practice, these programmes set both input requirements and include data collection of welfare outcome measures under the three key focus areas (see Table 7.1). Over time, we will be able to use these data to establish key areas of improvement and drive targeted interventions specific to our own supply chain. While not a new concept for researchers or veterinarians, creating opportunities for data-driven decisions about *animal welfare* in the retailer/food service space *is* relatively new, particularly for a company that does not own its food supply chain.

Table 7.1. Better Chicken.[a]

Better principle: broiler chickens	High level focus of principle in practice	Region[b]					
		Europe	Canada	USA	China	Australia	Rest of Asia Pacific
Better space[c]	Space available per animal			Further analysis required		Further analysis required	
	Thinning: removing a proportion of birds from the flock			N/A			
	Resources for the expression of natural behaviour			Further analysis required			
Better comfort[c]	Lighting: illumination and day length	>80% of stores during spring 2021	All stores spring 2021				
	Environmental conditions: ammonia, particulate matter, CO_2, litter quality, ventilation				All stores end of 2020		
Better health[c]	Flock health plan Health checks						
Better antibiotic stewardship[c,d]	Growth promotion and routine use						
Better manure management[e]	Storage and use of manure to avoid environmental pollution			All stores spring 2021		All stores end of 2020	All stores end of 2021

Continued

Table 7.1. Continued.

Better principle: broiler chickens	High level focus of principle in practice	Region[b]					
		Europe	Canada	USA	China	Australia	Rest of Asia Pacific
Better feed[e]	Non-deforestation feed						
Better monitoring[c]	Collection and reporting of welfare outcome measures						Further analysis required
Better future[c,d,e]	Non-deforestation feed						
	Highest priority critically important antibiotics for human health	2025	2025	2025	2025	2025	
	Pre-slaughter stunning method				Further analysis required		
	Genetic strain - bird type Natural light						

[a]Current as of 2020.
[b]The initial focus is on the largest regions NA, EU and AP – learnings will be used as input for implementation in remaining regions. 'Further analysis required' indicates the regional landscape is still being mapped, an action plan is being developed to close the gap or the system type is not a match for certain requirements (e.g. free range).
[c]Animal health and welfare principle.
[d]Public health principle.
[e]Environmental management principle.

7.2 Work and Life of a Corporate Sustainability Professional

The author joined IKEA in 2017 and works within the Health and Sustainability Team at IKEA Food. This team has specialists in various fields including human rights, climate and nutrition. Although her role is broader than animal welfare, she was primarily brought in because of her background in farm animal welfare science. That a multinational food company hired a full-time resource to focus on animal welfare is unique, as animal welfare is generally still a secondary topic, typically coming into consideration as it relates to brand risk, but not necessarily as an opportunity for enterprise growth. As such, it is often a component of other positions within quality, food safety or communications/brand management.

Her journey towards this role began in academia – her doctoral research focused on the element of choice, and its importance for dairy cattle welfare and production. After an initial experiment revealed choice as an opportunity to both allow animals to have what they want *and* improve yields (Motupalli *et al.*, 2014), it cemented the desire to place animal welfare within a larger context, potentially offering solutions for other complex sustainability issues. However, post-PhD, she felt that while opportunities to practically apply the science existed, it often got lost in journals and behind paywalls. She pursued animal welfare science not because she was drawn to the science itself, but because she saw a system that needed to evolve (for animals and humans alike) and science was a tool to enable that evolution.

So, she took a role with an NGO as a technical lead supporting their existing and developing food business partnerships. This decision came with risk – she was told by mentors that this role would jeopardize future job prospects owing to the contentious relationship between animal welfare NGOs and the agricultural industry. This input was jarring – she could be blacklisted even before her career had really started! She took the role anyway, challenging herself to merge science and advocacy effectively by seeking shared values between often divergent interests. While many of her existing industry relationships *did* change, that role offered her specific experience and a network which ultimately led to her current role within IKEA Food.

Applying the science in a role outside academia helped the author to develop the confidence to suggest a way forward when the path was murky, to become a generalist working with multiple species and to find common ground with those sharing opposing views in order to move the needle in favour of the *animal*. This work was also her first practical introduction to the impact food businesses could have on animal welfare with the right competence and vision.

7.3 Improving Animal Welfare as a Food Business

In her current role, she develops and supports the implementation of IKEA Food's sustainable sourcing strategy for the animal products in the food range across all of the 53 markets in which IKEA operates. In practice, this means her role is incredibly varied – she designs the agenda around animal welfare and how it fits into the larger sustainable agriculture space; works with internal and external stakeholders to refine and further this agenda; supports the development and maintenance of a basic governance structure to drive the agenda and ensure accountability; provides the knowledge base for practical implementation; and represents the agenda publicly. The most important function she serves, however, is to empower *others* to drive this agenda within the business. The ultimate win being that one day, she is not actually needed because the topic is deeply embedded within normal business operations.

7.3.1 Empowering non-experts within a food business to drive an animal welfare agenda

In the author's experience, commercial animal production is a knowledge gap for many people in food businesses and it is not yet common knowledge that animal welfare is a scientific field with measurable parameters. As a result, much of her initial work has been to raise awareness of the topic across the whole company – *what* it is, *why* we should care, what we can *do* about it and, more importantly, what do we *want* to do about it? The focus has also been on arming individuals with the tools they need to implement the agenda, empowering them to make changes themselves, as discussed in Chapters 2 and 4. This has been via multiple mediums:

- Presentations and workshops for varying levels of management: animal welfare basics including production cycles, prioritization of welfare issues, wider benefits and mitigation solutions.
- Practice guidelines and implementation support documents: individual species requirements and their evidence base. These are key for non-experts to engage with suppliers successfully and confidently, as they provide the necessary level of knowledge to have meaningful and *critical* conversations.
- Technical training sessions: practical assessment of the BPs on the ground, particularly when evaluating new suppliers. Understanding the right questions to ask, how to frame those questions to get the information you need and the importance of direct animal observation.
- Internal case studies capturing value for human and animal stakeholders alike: documenting and sharing evidence that the food business is driving forward a beneficial agenda for multiple stakeholders. This strengthens both morale and resolve as something that might have once felt abstract is now tangible and accessible. It also creates meaningful opportunities for engagement with suppliers on specific constraints and support needs – giving us a real-time reality check, and an opportunity to work in a more agile way.

Taken together, the author hopes that over time these approaches will empower everyone within the business, even those who are not subject-matter experts, to effectively move the agenda forward. Some success has become evident as two species BPs are currently embedded in internal supply chain processes and are moving forward with limited expert intervention.

Case Study 2: Capturing the Supplier Perspective

A regional pilot study examining supplier perception of IKEA Better Chicken barns compared with a more conventional barn set-up revealed that animal welfare-focused criteria appeared to both improve bird welfare and enable a better working environment for humans. Opinions were captured from all levels of staff (barn workers, the company veterinarian and management) and the general perception was that the criteria improved bird welfare by allowing them to express natural behaviour as well as reduce severity of painful health conditions like footpad dermatitis. There was also a perceived benefit to the increased space allowance – it was noted that birds could better access feed and water, which stakeholders felt allowed the birds to grow better. Beyond this, there was a clear recognition from the barn workers' point of view that the IKEA barns made their working environment 'more comfortable' with specific reference to brighter lighting, improved air quality and opportunities to watch birds 'play' via the provision of environmental enrichment. Watching birds 'enjoy themselves' through 'play' was noted as an experience that made individual workers feel 'relaxed'.

Shifting Perspectives: The Power of Being on the Ground

For most food businesses, procurement teams are key partners for successfully improving animal welfare in a supply chain. Procurement teams often have expertise in cost optimization, product quality and broad knowledge related to further processing (how a raw material becomes a finished product like a meatball) but may have limited knowledge on processing or animal production. Ensuring that procurement professionals within your company are empowered to confidently take on an animal welfare agenda themselves is a precondition for success. Some concrete steps and general advice to support an animal welfare practitioner currently on this journey are outlined in the following text.

- Start with the assumption that people generally want to support an agenda related to a more sustainable future.

The battle is not about getting people to care, it's about providing them a meaningful way to contribute in their specific functional role, recognizing the constraints of their function.

- Create opportunities for on-the-ground visits with yourself or other animal welfare practitioners.

Farm and slaughterhouse visits have been one of the most important forms of engagement on the topic of animal welfare for IKEA Food. They have enabled

Continued

Continued.

procurement professionals who may not have previously had occasion to connect the finished product (meatball, chicken fillet etc.) with the animal *itself* to find a more personal connection to the animal welfare agenda, as well as the BPs as a whole. These visits also create a space for them to ask critical questions at the source. Most importantly, it inspired a few to see what *could* be if we didn't simply accept the status quo.

Example 1

While examining foot injuries during a broiler farm visit (Fig. 7.2), a member of the procurement team was visibly upset when the author identified severely lame birds unable to walk. The individual shared with the author that it was sad and wanted to know what could be done about it. The author connected criteria within the existing animal welfare agenda including stocking density, genetic strain, environmental enrichment and welfare outcome measures to this individual bird and her lameness status in real time. By doing so, this individual was able to form a more practical and personal connection to the animal welfare agenda and felt emboldened to drive this work forward in the supply chain.

Example 2

When reflecting on a series of farm visits during the initial development of the BPs, a senior leader in procurement shared that they 'didn't know what was possible', and that these visits were the single most important part of their journey to getting on board with the animal welfare agenda. They shared that imagining a different way can be difficult, but seeing that many producers are already farming differently helps make the vision more realistic.

- Keep the pre-visit preparation simple.

Share the basics around animal needs and wants so they feel confident enough to ask questions on-site at the farm. However, do not overwhelm them with knowledge – allow them the space to discover for themselves whether or not their on-farm experience matches their own expectations and values. Encourage exploration and curiosity – ask them what they feel is positive and what they might do differently. During these discussions it often becomes clear that their expectations are already linked to the BPs approach.

- De-brief post-visit.

Make sure to cement the connections between the on-farm experience and the animal welfare agenda. Ideally after this experience they should be able to speak on the basics of the agenda themselves with conviction, pride and a more personal connection.

Continued.

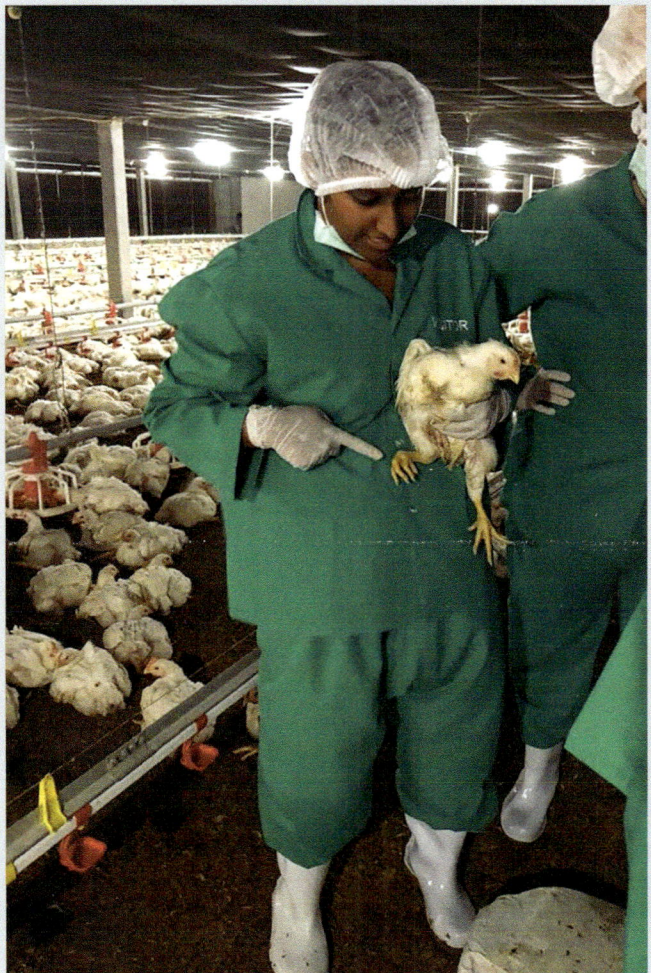

Fig. 7.2. Identification and discussion of foot health problems in broiler chickens during a practical training session with key internal stakeholders. (© P. Motupalli.)

- Create opportunities for enjoyment!

Learning about animals is fun! Most people can naturally connect with our science if opportunities are provided (Fig. 7.3). Scientists are also human – sharing an emotional investment in this topic does not weaken the science, rather it inspires others and forges connections.

Continued

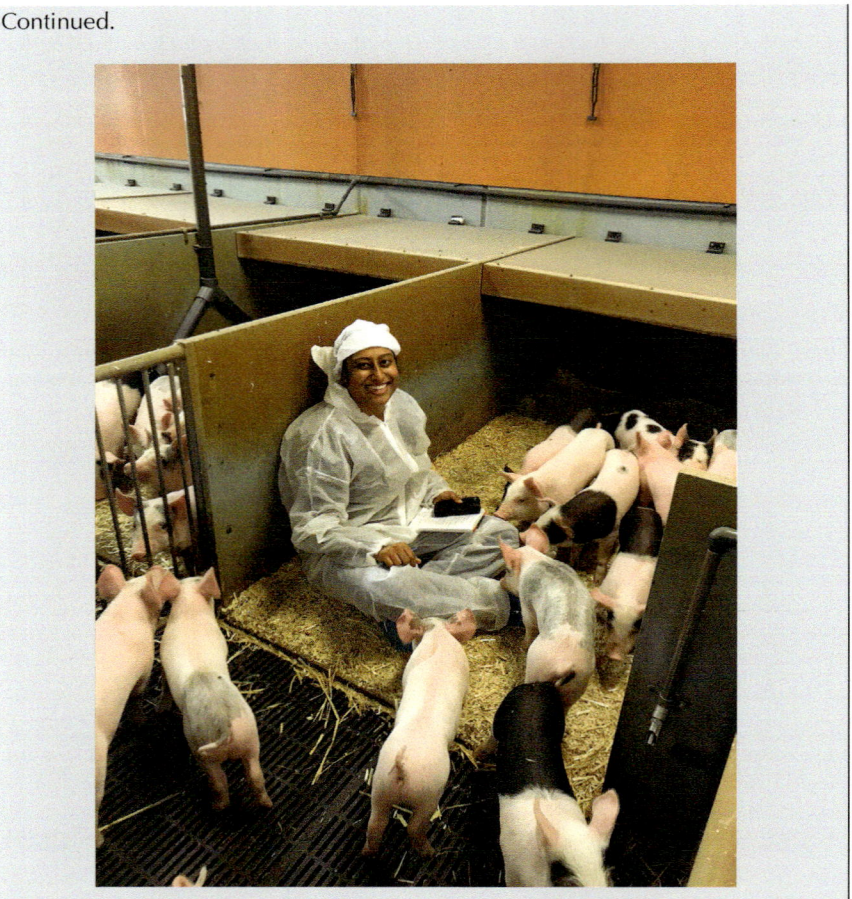

Continued.

Fig. 7.3. Testing the application of humans as novel enrichment for young pigs during an on-farm training session with key internal stakeholders. (© P. Motupalli.)

7.4 Overcoming Challenges

Acting as a change agent within an established food business is both exhilarating and frustrating. There is opportunity for enormous impact, with smart, innovative solutions-focused people and inspiring leadership. Yet, progress is often slow, conventional methods are the norm, and depending on what level your business sits at in the overall supply chain you may not be set up to make the change you really want to make. Three specific challenges are outlined in the following text with some of the solutions that IKEA Food is exploring.

Challenge 1: IKEA is a low-cost retailer and prides itself on affordability by driving supply chain efficiencies that continually reduce costs for the customer.

Short term, the BPs will have a cost impact. Moving away from caged systems, rethinking genetics and reducing stocking densities are clear cost drivers. It is difficult to take on this cost impact as a business when there is not a huge precedent yet for broad, established benefits related to animal welfare specifically.

Potential solutions: First, IKEA Food is attempting to shift the mindset within the business about what an animal-based raw material *should* cost. Better Chicken, Better Pig, etc. is the new baseline for the raw material cost. Whatever the business was getting before is not comparable material. Second, the business is investigating how to better utilize carcasses across the range globally. Even small changes like buying chicken leg meat with the skin *on* versus buying those materials separately have cost-saving potential. Third, our data collection requirements in the BPs will allow for better insights into how improvements in animal health can have a positive impact on long-term costs.

Challenge 2: In general, if a food company does not make up the majority of business for an individual supplier, there is limited leverage to influence change. Even when suppliers *can* meet the BPs targets without changing their existing production methods, there is no guarantee that they are optimal related to other business needs – quality, raw material type, appropriate volumes, compliance with our supplier code of conduct, food safety, geography, etc.

Potential solutions: Engagement in a number of multi-stakeholder initiatives to collectively drive progress across the whole industry. For example, IKEA is a founding member of the Global Coalition for Animal Welfare, the first business-led collective dedicated to improving welfare in global food supply chains. It also sits on the Aquaculture Stewardship Council technical working group on animal welfare, broadening the scope of a standard widely used across the seafood industry. Aside from external efforts, the business is also in the process of consolidating its supply chain and range – this will enable optimization of total purchase volumes to increase purchasing power and enable more flexibility for creating strategic supplier partnerships that can further the sustainability agenda.

Challenge 3: It is generally postulated that improving animal welfare beyond physical health will negatively impact carbon emissions owing to creating a more inefficient system (efficiency in this context means maximizing outputs while minimizing inputs).

Potential solutions: First, the leadership driving IKEA's climate agenda recognizes that solutions we propose to achieve the goal of becoming Climate Positive (sequestering more carbon than we emit) by 2030 should not generate negative externalities elsewhere (e.g. human rights, animal welfare). This sets a tone where the focus is on mitigating trade-offs rather than being held back by them. Second, the business is attempting to learn from industry players who have managed carbon-neutral, high-welfare production via a combination of alternative feed sources (removing the climate impact from land-use change), renewable energy and alternative waste streams (circular agriculture), but all of this has yet to be measured properly over time and at scale. IKEA Food is also learning from the 'regenerative agriculture' space with ruminant production –

trying to understand the scalable opportunities for livestock production to contribute to the climate agenda (carbon capture, biodiversity, livelihoods). Third, optimizing the balance of proteins from both plant and animal sources within our range portfolio may allow us to continue to push the boundaries for low-cost retailers in the animal welfare space while still mitigating our emissions at the ingredient level.

More generally, the holistic nature of the BPs, in particular the environmental management pillar, should allow for some level of mitigation related to impact created by the animal welfare pillar. There is also hope that over time, the BPs will improve mortality rates and impact quality and yield leading to less wastage.

Much of this is exploratory even if backed by clear reasoning however, and IKEA Food is still in the early stages of implementation. It is not yet clear what the impact of the proposed mitigation strategies will be, or if it will be enough to make the trade-offs acceptable. Standing still is not really an option however, and the organization reasonably believes this is the right direction, given the multiple avenues it is exploring for mitigation.

7.5 Conclusions and Future Direction

The integration of an animal welfare strategy within a food business is a long game. It starts with a foundation of animal welfare science frameworks, recognizing that allowing animals to express natural behaviour and providing opportunities for positive experiences resonates strongly with non-experts. It then becomes a stakeholder engagement task, empowering non-specialists to take on the agenda by creating personal and tangible connections to the impact of the agenda.

Although emerging evidence suggests that a focus on animal welfare can help drive solutions for broader sustainability challenges, animals are often an overlooked stakeholder. Future opportunities to ensure that animal welfare remains a focus area within a food business lie with continuing to identify ways that improving animal welfare can contribute to more resilient supply chains capable of withstanding system shocks (ASF, climate change, etc.) in the long term.

The expertise gap of animal welfare inside businesses offers an interesting niche for recent graduates to find roles outside of academia, where they can actively apply their scientific training to help businesses drive the agenda from within.

7.6 Recommended Resources

- IKEA People and Planet Positive Sustainability Strategy, https://preview.thenewsmarket.com/Previews/IKEA/DocumentAssets/511938_v3.PDF (accessed 7 April 2021).

- IKEA More sustainable agriculture and better animal welfare, https://about.ikea.com/en/about-us/our-view-on/more-sustainable-animal-agriculture-and-better-animal-welfare (accessed 22 April 2021).
- FAI Farms, https://www.faifarms.com (accessed 7 April 2021).
- Global Coalition for Animal Welfare, www.gc-animalwelfare.org (accessed 7 April 2021).
- Aquaculture Stewardship Council Technical Working Group on Fish Welfare, https://www.asc-aqua.org/weve-been-working-hard-on-new-fish-welfare-requirements-heres-the-latest (accessed 7 April 2021).

Acknowledgements

The author is grateful to Beth Ventura, Freyja Frímannsdóttir and Seetaram Motupalli for their review of an earlier version of this chapter and to IKEA Food for being the little rebel within a home furnishing business.

References

Brown, S.M., Bush, S.J., Summers, K.M., Hume, D.A. and Lawrence, A.B. (2018) Environmental enriched pigs have transcriptional profiles consistent with neuroprotective effects and reduced microglial activity. *Behavioural Brain Research* 350, 6–15.

Bradsher, K. and Tang, A. (2019) China responds slowly and a pig disease becomes a lethal epidemic. *The New York Times*. Available at: https://www.nytimes.com/2019/12/17/business/china-pigs-african-swine-fever.html (accessed 1 August 2020).

Dawkins, M. (2019) Animal welfare as preventative medicine. *Animal Welfare* 28, 137–141.

Fraser, D., Weary, D.M., Pajor, E.A. and Milligan, B.N. (1997) A scientific conception of animal welfare that reflects ethical concerns. *Animal Welfare* 6, 187–205.

International Panel on Climate Change (IPCC) (2019) Climate change and land: An IPCC special report on climate change, desertification, sustainable land management, food security, and greenhouse gas fluxes in terrestrial ecosystems. Available at: https://www.ipcc.ch/srccl (accessed 1 August 2020).

Mellor, D.J. (2017) Operational details of the Five Domains Model and its key applications to the assessment and management of animal welfare. *Animals* 7, 60.

Motupalli, P.M., Sinclair, L.A., Charlton, G.L., Bleach, E.A. and Rutter, S.M. (2014) Preference and behavior of lactating dairy cows given free access to pasture at two herbage masses and two distances. *Journal of Animal Science* 92, 5175–5184. https://doi.org/10.2527/jas.2014-8046

O'Neill, J. (2015) Antimicrobials in Agriculture and the Environment: Reducing Unnecessary Waste. Available at https://amr-review.org/Publications.html (accessed 1 July 2020).

Organisation for Economic Co-operation and Development (OECD) (2020) Building back better: A sustainable resilient recovery after COVID-19. Available at: www.oecd.org/coronavirus/policy-responses/building-back-better-a-sustainable-resilient-recovery-after-covid-19-52b869f5 (accessed 1 August 2020).

Rault, J.L., Hintze, S., Camerlink, I. and Yee, J.R. (2020) Positive welfare and the like: Distinct views and a proposed framework. *Frontiers in Veterinary Science* 7, 370.

Tatemoto, P., Bernardino, T., Alves, L., de Oliveira Souza, A.C., Palme, R. and Zanella, A.J. (2019) Environmental enrichment for pregnant sows modulates HPA-axis and behavior in the offspring. *Applied Animal Behaviour Science* 220, 104854.

United Nations Environment Programme (UNEP) (2020) Preventing the next pandemic – Zoonotic diseases and how to break the chain of transmission. Available at: https://www.unenvironment.org/resources/report/preventing-future-zoonotic-disease-outbreaks-protecting-environment-animals-and (accessed 12 August 2020).

Van Dixhoorn, I.D.E., Reimert, I., Middelkoop, J., Bolhuis, J.E., Wisselink, H.J. *et al.* (2016) Enriched housing reduces disease susceptibility to co-infection with porcine reproductive and respiratory virus (PRRSV) and *Actinobacillu spleuropneumoniae* (*A. pleuropneumoniae*) in young pigs. *PLoS ONE* 11. https://doi.org/10.1371/journal.pone.0161832

Ventura, B.A., von Keyserlingk, M.A.G., Wittman, H. and Weary, D.M. (2016) What difference does a visit make? Changes in animal welfare perceptions after interested citizens tour a dairy farm. *PLoS ONE* 11. https://doi.org/10.1371/journal.pone.0154733

World Organisation for Animal Health (OIE) (2020) Global situation of African swine fever. Available at: https://www.oie.int/fileadmin/Home/eng/Animal_Health_in_the_World/docs/pdf/Disease_cards/ASF/Report_47_Global_situation_ASF.pdf (accessed 1 August 2020).

8 Farm Animal Welfare in the Nigerian context

Mabel Aworh-Ajumobi
Department of Veterinary and Pest Control Services, Federal Ministry of Agriculture and Rural Development, Abuja, Nigeria

8.1 Introduction

The average Nigerian person on the street cannot relate to the term 'animal welfare' because this is a relatively new theme in their society. Nigeria, being the most populous black nation, has great cultural diversity, customs, traditions and over 250 ethnic groups (CIA, 2020). People see animals as beasts of burden or as a means of livelihood, especially since farm animals are raised for food and eventually are sold to provide income. Animals such as dogs that are companion animals in other cultures are often farmed for food among Efik people in southern Nigeria, and therefore end up on the table as these cultures consider them to be special delicacies, or useful for medicinal purposes. However, the wealthy do not have the same ideology and are willing to spend whatever it takes to ensure the welfare of their pets or companion animals.

Farm animal welfare, which combines animal husbandry, health and behaviour, means raising animals humanely in an environment where they can behave naturally hence using less feed, fuel and water as characteristics of a less intensive farming system (World Animal Protection, 2020). Farm animals such as chickens, pigs, goats, sheep, cattle, camels, donkeys and rabbits are considered an integral part of the human community because people depend on these animals for food, labour, entertainment, transportation, sports and research. Donkeys and horses are mainly considered as working animals; however, in some cultures they are raised with other farm animals for food. In some communities, people live in close proximity to their animals, which are considered part of their everyday life. Although these farm animals are very important to people, very little attention is paid to their welfare, in terms of nutrition, shelter, healthcare and their environment. People often do not relate to animals as sentient beings with the ability to experience pain and discomfort (Proctor *et al.*, 2013). These animals often experience discomfort during different aspects of production, such as during transportation from one location to the other, or during routine husbandry procedures owing to stress from handling. In some instances shelter, an integral aspect of welfare, is not provided, exposing farm animals to very harsh weather conditions. Nigeria has a tropical climate with two major seasons. The wet (rainy) season is usually from April to October and prone to flooding, especially in riverine communities. The dry season is from November to March. In most cases, farm animals are reared outdoors in an extensive system allowing the freedom to express their natural behaviour, although some farm animals are reared indoors in an intensive system. In some scenarios, especially among the Fulani nomads, animals are allowed to roam about in search of basic needs such as food and water allowing them the freedom to express their natural behaviours. In other instances, these animals fall ill because they lack appropriate shelter as well as good-quality diets. Poor handling of farm animals can be observed, such as when a farmer is seen to hit the animals (cattle, sheep and goats) with sticks in an attempt to facilitate movement, as opposed to gentle handling methods that are devoid of pain and discomfort.

Animal welfare is an upcoming theme in Nigeria and has to date not been given due consideration by national or international non-governmental organizations (NGOs) owing to their very limited presence in the country. In other African countries where animal welfare has been embraced by the people, the presence of NGOs such as Donkey Sanctuary, World Animal Protection, the International Coalition for Farm Animal Welfare (ICFAW), etc. has positively influenced good animal welfare practices. The average person on the streets who is struggling to afford their daily meals finds it very difficult to provide their animals with the basic needs of food, water, shelter, good transportation and healthcare. In some rural communities, farmers cannot afford the services of a veterinarian to provide healthcare for their animals. Veterinary care is often only accessible to the wealthy and a small proportion of others who understand the importance of veterinary services. This forces farmers to purchase drugs over the counter and administer them to the animals themselves, which endangers the lives of their animals, who may receive the wrong medication, an overdose or the wrong method of administration.

Case Study 1: Better Welfare Practices for Polo Horses

Horses used for sporting activities such as polo horses in Nigeria enjoy better animal welfare than farm animals, although they have limited ability to express their natural behaviour as they are usually in the stables most of the time. This is largely because the wealthy owners listen to the recommendations provided by their veterinarians to ensure better welfare for the horses. These horses have very good housing, food and healthcare, and are usually transported following the recommendations provided by the World Organisation for Animal Health (OIE) for equids. Horses used for polo are very expensive and owners want their animals to perform optimally, hence they are willing to follow all of the recommendations to ensure that their animals perform exceptionally at the games. Financial resources and education are key to achieving good farm animal welfare practices in Nigeria and other developing economies.

8.2 Work and Life as an Animal Welfare Practitioner

In Nigeria, Dr Aworh-Ajumobi works as a government veterinarian at the Federal Ministry of Agriculture and Rural Development in Abuja. The OIE has developed a number of animal welfare standards and guidelines for member countries, and these have been adopted for use in Nigeria. The author is Nigeria's OIE national focal point for animal welfare, and works under the directive of the OIE delegate for Nigeria – the Chief Veterinary Officer of Nigeria and Director of the Department of Veterinary and Pest Control Services in the Federal Ministry of Agriculture and Rural Development, Abuja. Animal welfare activities fall directly under his jurisdiction and the author assists him in handling animal welfare-related tasks.

Nigeria has an animal welfare strategy approved by the National Council on Agriculture and Rural Development, which provides the policy direction on animal welfare issues for the country. Nigeria's animal welfare strategy has the following vision: 'A nation where the welfare of animals is respected, promoted and advanced, simultaneously with the pursuit of progress and socio-economic development'. Nigeria has an animal welfare consultative committee made up of key stakeholders who meet every 3 years to revise the animal welfare strategy, which guides the implementation of animal welfare-related activities. The current animal diseases legislation has been revised to include a chapter on animal welfare, as this is required to provide the legal framework for animal welfare-related work and activities. One of the responsibilities of the Department of Veterinary and Pest Control Services is to develop animal welfare policy, as well as standards, for the implementation of animal welfare activities. In addition, the Department's responsibilities involve awareness creation on animal welfare using various platforms such as workshops, stakeholders' engagement, and the use of information, education and communication materials to sensitize the general public.

The priorities of the Nigerian animal welfare strategy include:

- Developing national animal welfare standards, including broad consultation of industry, NGOs, etc.
- Raising awareness at national, sub-national and district levels of the importance of complying with animal welfare standards.
- Improving the participation of all stakeholders in compliance with national animal welfare standards.

The OIE, in addition to developing animal welfare standards, also provides regular training for animal welfare focal points and this has helped the author in carrying out her responsibilities in relation to farm animal welfare. For example, she had the opportunity to make a presentation entitled 'Challenges for the implementation of animal welfare standards at national level' at a regional OIE seminar for focal points in Lesotho, 2018. The talk was presented to OIE focal points from different countries in the African region and was a forum to share animal welfare experiences from developing economies to learn from those who have got it right. Some focal points at the training could relate to the author's talk as they had the same experience in their respective countries.

> **Case Study 2: Training Farmers on Good Animal Welfare Practices**
>
> Dr Mabel Aworh-Ajumobi had the opportunity to organize a workshop on behalf of the Department of Veterinary and Pest Control Services on good farm animal welfare practices among several stakeholders: poultry farmers, cattle farmers, pig farmers, sheep and goat farmers as well as chicken sellers, representatives of farm animal transporters, slaughterhouse workers, private and government veterinarians and regulatory bodies in the food animal industry in Abuja, Nigeria's capital city, in January 2018. The participants at the workshop were diverse, especially in terms of their level of education. This informed the author's choice of workshop presentations ranging from PowerPoint slides, use of flip charts, role-play and visuals particularly videos. The well-educated participants appreciated the use of PowerPoint slides as well as flip charts for the delivery of the workshop training. Those who had minimal education found the PowerPoint slides and flip charts very boring and did not get the key messages being passed across to them. They were super excited to see the OIE cattle welfare demonstration video at the end, and they were then able to appreciate the message the author was trying to communicate earlier using the slides and flip charts. The author also found the use of working in smaller groups very effective in passing on her message. This method was useful in identifying the different voices among the study participants to make sure that everyone was being carried along and it helped her to meet their varied
>
>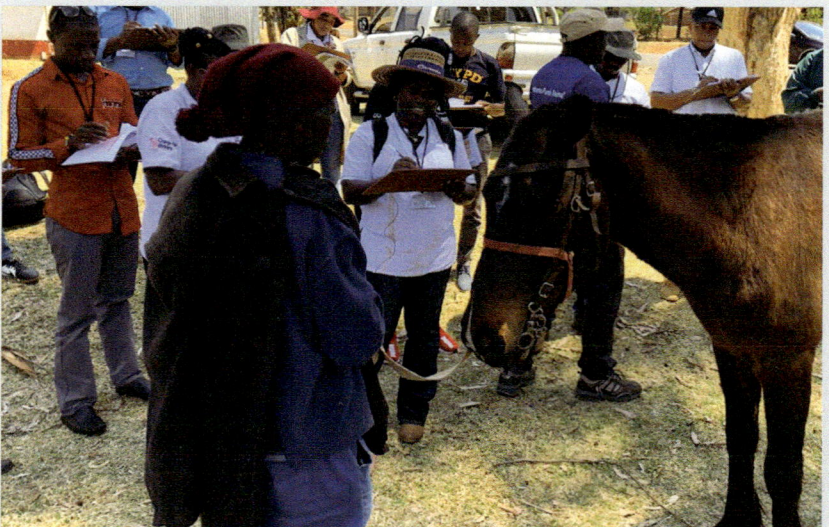
>
> **Fig. 8.1.** The author assessing the welfare of working equids.

> **Case Study 2:** Continued.
> expectations. At the end of the workshop, pig farmers and poultry farmers requested animal welfare demonstration videos to address the other species of farm animals. Unfortunately, Dr Aworh-Ajumobi had not seen OIE welfare demonstration videos for other farm animals.
> It is important to perform an audience analysis prior to organizing any training on animal welfare. Sometimes, practical hands-on demonstration sessions on the farm with live animals are important for effective communication. At an OIE training session in Lesotho, Dr Aworh-Ajumobi had the opportunity to participate in hands-on assessment of equine welfare (Fig. 8.1). This made it very easy for her to comprehend what the instructors had said while in class. Hands-on practical sessions make it easier for the audience to comprehend and will help in driving home the key messages more than just talking or using slides.

Previously the author trained as a veterinarian in Nigeria, however she is currently undertaking a PhD programme alongside her work as Nigeria's OIE focal point on animal welfare. Dr Aworh-Ajumobi has had the opportunity to engage with professional societies such as the International Society for Applied Ethology (ISAE) to learn about animal welfare from other countries and (as of 2021) is currently the ISAE country liaison for Nigeria. She has had the opportunity to meet stakeholders on animal welfare from different countries and successfully coordinated the ISAE Global Virtual Meeting 2020 for Africa–Central Asia–Middle East in August. There have been successful connections with other key welfare officials from the Middle East since the meeting.

8.3 Improving Animal Welfare as a Government

Animal welfare in Nigeria, like in many other low- and middle-income countries has been poorly defined and regulated. Welfare problems are enormous; however, one key issue impeding the welfare of farm animals in Nigeria is the minimal presence of animal welfare international NGOs and civil society groups. Nigeria, being the most populous black nation, is currently making efforts to develop animal welfare legislation to ensure that the welfare of animals, including farm animals, improves. The presence of animal welfare NGOs in Nigeria would complement the efforts of the government to ensure animals have better welfare. The roles of animal welfare NGOs cannot be overemphasized, as their presence makes it easier to implement government animal welfare policies, by supporting the development of appropriate animal welfare legislation and organizing educational campaigns geared towards changes in human perspectives on providing basic welfare needs for farm animals (Wilkins et al., 2005).

Other challenges include the paucity of funds for animal welfare activities, as this is not considered a priority. Limited financial resources for animal welfare work have made it difficult to create much-needed awareness especially among the target group of farmers. Many farmers are unaware of animal welfare principles; others have some level of knowledge but a lack of financial resources has deterred them from providing the basic welfare needs for their farm animals. Many farmers involved in rearing farm animals lack formal education and find it difficult to understand key animal welfare concepts.

One important welfare issue that keeps reoccurring is the slaughter of pregnant animals at the abattoir for food, although most farmers claim that they were not aware that their animals were pregnant (Fayemi and Muchenje, 2013). Animal health is an integral component of animal welfare: a happy animal is a healthy animal. Violating any aspect of the five domains of animal welfare results in a state of ill health. Evidence has shown that farm animals are able to communicate their feelings with the farmer using their vocal sounds, for example (Adesokan Lawal-Adebowale, 2020); however, it needs a knowledgeable farmer to understand what their animals are trying to communicate.

The lack of availability of species-specific animal welfare training videos for practical demonstrations of basic animal welfare principles to educate farmers on how best to ensure that farm animals receive better care has further compounded the issue of poor animal welfare practices. The OIE has developed a few videos for these purposes, particularly for cattle welfare; however, there is the need to ensure that such videos are available for other species of animals in very simple language. It is easier to communicate with those with little formal education using such training videos, especially for the purpose of behavioural change.

Poor animal welfare is evident at the various stages of farm animal husbandry in Nigeria, ranging from inappropriate housing to inadequate floor spacing per animal, to poor or malnourished diets, as well as poor waste management on farms (Dixon *et al.*, 2001). Other welfare problems have been observed during the transportation of farm animals, at holdings in the livestock market and slaughter facilities. Primitive and crude methods are still being employed for transporting animals, such as transporting a camel in the trunk of a car (Fig. 8.2).

Sometimes livestock are overburdened, causing pain (Fig. 8.3), or are transported in overcrowded trucks (Fig. 8.4), resulting in lameness on arrival at the markets. Chickens are often seen tied upside down when transported using motor bikes as opposed to the use of crates. This would cause them poor welfare owing to fear, distress or injured hocks. This situation is fast improving owing to government interventions targeting awareness creation of the proper means to transport chickens, devoid of pain and discomfort.

Farm animals are also observed to experience pain during slaughter owing to the rough manner in which they are handled. While animals are being slaughtered, other animals awaiting slaughter are allowed to watch the painful process their fellow animals being slaughtered have to go through.

Farm Animal Welfare in the Nigerian Context 119

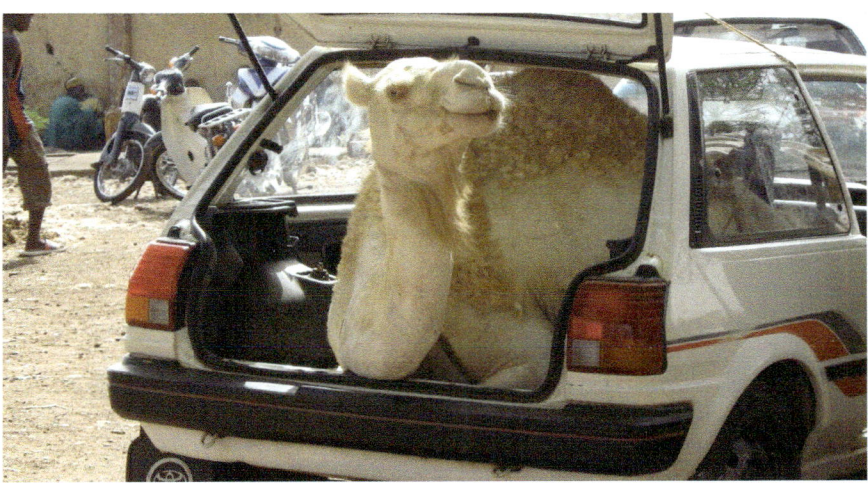

Fig. 8.2. A camel in the trunk of a car, showing welfare issues during transport. (Photo: Professor Garba Sharubutu, Animal Welfare Initiative.)

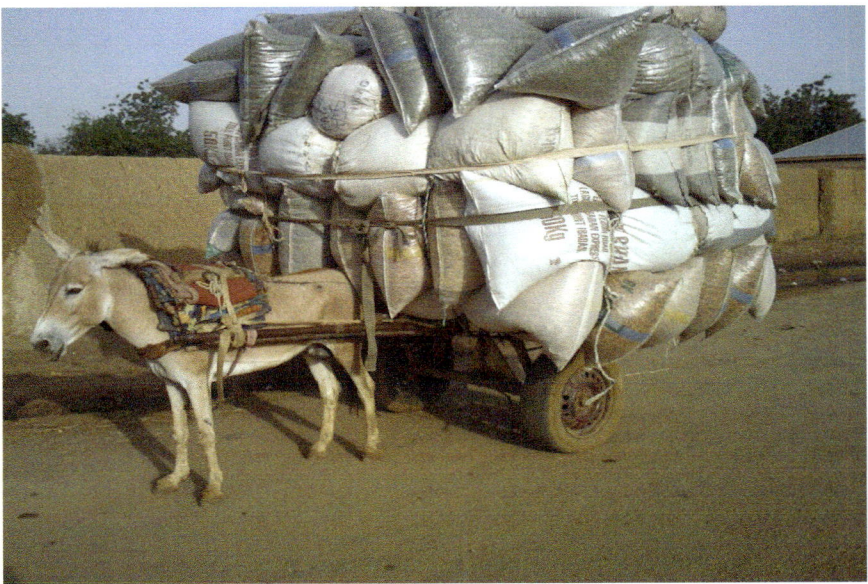

Fig. 8.3. Donkey overburdened with excessive load because of human behaviour. The donkey has been made to carry several heavy bags of grain, which inflicted wounds causing it pain. Back wounds were observed after the load was taken off. (Photo: Professor Garba Sharubutu, Animal Welfare Initiative.)

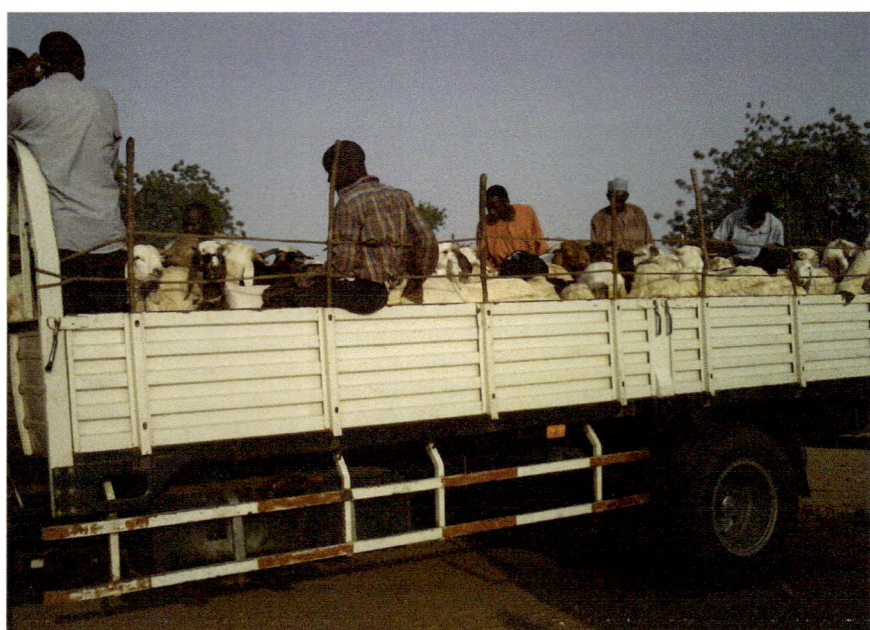

Fig. 8.4. Transporting sheep and goats in overcrowded truck. (Photo: Professor Sharubutu, Animal Welfare Initiative.)

Stunning before slaughter, as recommended by the OIE, has not been accepted in Nigeria owing to cultural and religious beliefs that do not allow slaughter of an unconscious animal, therefore resulting in the use of crude methods that inflict unnecessary pain on the animals at slaughter. It is a common practice for workers at a slaughterhouse to twist the tail of a cow in an attempt to forcefully get it to move prior to being restrained just before slaughter. Twisting the tail of the cow to facilitate movement is painful and should be discouraged. On arrival at the slaughter area, the cow's four legs are tied together. In trying to address welfare issues, the OIE has made recommendations for the slaughter of farm animals without causing undue stress, pain and discomfort to the animals (OIE, 2019). These OIE recommendations have been adopted by the country, although they have not been enforced nationwide.

Although animals are viewed as either beasts of burden or sources of food and income, the pastoralist can sacrifice all they have to preserve their animals. Certain cultures take delight in raising farm animals as part of the family unit, so much so that they eventually become emotionally attached to them. In such communities, children are made to walk the animals for long distances in search of green pasture. Farm animals in the city, particularly cattle, are often seen walking very long distances in search of food and water (see Fig. 8.5). Other farm animals, such as sheep and goats, are allowed to roam freely in

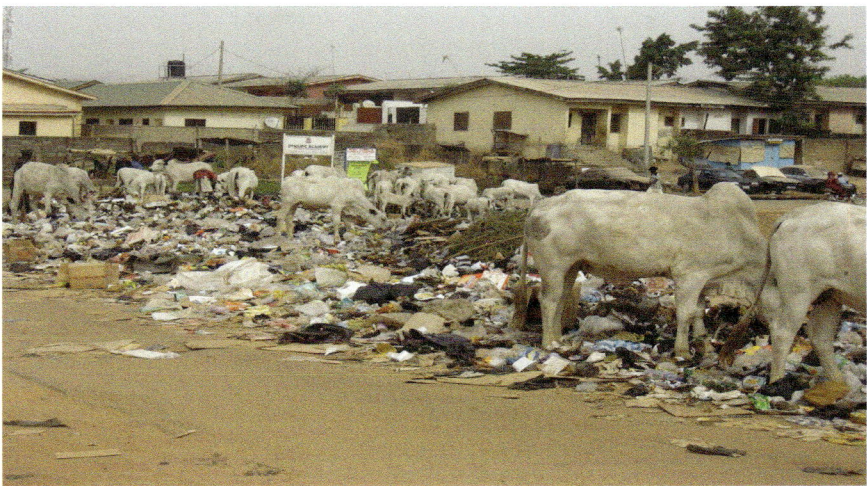

Fig. 8.5. Cattle feeding on a refuse dump. (Photo: Professor Garba Sharubutu, Animal Welfare Initiative.)

search of food and water exposing them to all sorts of danger, including harsh weather conditions, road accidents, as well as poor diet.

Illiteracy and poverty have also made matters worse, especially in seeking healthcare for sick animals. In some instances, farmers have to administer drugs to the animals by themselves, which runs the risk of them not adhering to the correct dosage, using the wrong route of administration or maybe even administering the wrong drugs.

8.4 Overcoming Challenges

One of the biggest barriers to change is human behaviour. Once a person has cultivated the wrong habits or ways of doing certain things, it becomes very difficult to get them to change their behaviour. The attitude of some people towards farm animals is based on their limited knowledge of animal welfare, as they cannot relate to the fact that animals are sentient beings and do feel pain.

The legislation is very important when introducing new concepts as it provides the legal framework for its implementation. The process of developing legislation requires time and resources, which are not readily available. In Nigeria, there is the animal welfare strategy that provides the country with policy direction regarding welfare issues. The current legislation, which provides some legal framework for animal welfare, has obsolete fines and penalties; therefore, it has been revised to include a detailed chapter on animal welfare. The process of getting the revised legislation approved requires enormous amounts of time and resources. It is not certain when the revised legislation will be approved and signed into law.

Behavioural change communication can be achieved using practical demonstrations or training videos on animal welfare concepts. Training and retraining of farmers are necessary to achieve behavioural change. In Nigeria, good animal welfare practices have been communicated effectively to farmers using the OIE video for cattle welfare, because the stakeholders at the training preferred video to PowerPoint presentation. Using role models such as community leaders or religious leaders as agents of change in communicating the desired behavioural change can be explored. This has been explored in Nigeria, although not in connection with animal welfare but in addressing important public health issues, such as eradicating polio. Involving international animal welfare NGOs can complement government efforts with animal welfare initiatives. Learning from the experiences of other African countries, international animal welfare NGOs made it possible to establish animal welfare legislation in Kenya. Funds are key to implementing good farm animal welfare; hence, it is important to have dedicated budget lines for animal welfare activities at the government level.

The animal welfare strategy document is currently used to guide the implementation of farm animal welfare in Nigeria. The revised legislation required to provide the legal framework for the implementation of animal welfare standards nationwide is a work in progress. The involvement of international animal welfare organizations will be instrumental to the implementation of good farm animal welfare practices in the country; for example, by facilitating educational campaigns, public awareness geared towards animal welfare legislation and so on. These NGOs when present will complement the efforts of the government in addressing farm animal welfare issues. Development of more species-specific practical demonstration videos on good farm animal welfare practices will be useful for behavioural change communication. The Nigerian government needs help in achieving these, owing to the paucity of funds as well as the required expertise.

How to Change the Behaviour of Cattle Farmers in Nigeria and Other African Countries

The following text describes how you can put practical steps in place to actually change farmers' behaviour from using a stick to hit an animal to using flags to guide them when trying to compel the animals to move in a certain direction.

- Step 1: Identify the group of people who need to change. Study the cattle farmers to observe what they know about animal welfare and the reason for the behaviour you are trying to change.
- Step 2: Praise them for what they are doing right. Encourage good animal welfare practices you have observed by acknowledging what they are doing correctly and provide rewards.

Continued

Continued.

- Step 3: Use videos to provide practical tips on good farm animal welfare. For example, use the OIE video on cattle welfare to provide practical tips on good welfare practices.
- Step 4: Obtain feedback from the farmers on other areas where they are willing to change their behaviour.
- Step 5: Focus on the behaviour that the farmers are willing to change, then retrain, such as by using the OIE video on cattle welfare.
- Step 6: Training and retraining are essential until they have mastered this new behaviour.

8.5 Conclusions

In the interim, while awaiting the signing of the revised legislation that provides a legal framework for animal welfare activities in Nigeria, awareness creation as well as education of farmers towards behavioural change can be embarked upon. This will facilitate the implementation of animal welfare policy as well as good farm animal welfare practices. The list that follows itemizes the main concerns and recommendations to progress farm animal welfare in Nigeria.

- Farm animals largely undergo suffering owing to malnutrition, overloading of work animals and ill-treatment of food animals. Draught animals are usually exploited for farm work. Cruelty to farm animals occurs at every stage before slaughter and during slaughter.
- Farm animals, particularly cattle, travelling for slaughter are made to walk long distances or transported in overcrowded trucks and usually arrive at the slaughter facilities either lame or seriously injured.
- Stunning prior to slaughter has not been accepted and therefore is not being practised in Nigeria owing to cultural and religious beliefs.
- The OIE Guidelines/Standards on Animal Welfare have been adopted by Nigeria, although this is yet to be implemented nationwide. Motivating people towards good animal welfare practices is a challenge in low-resource settings where poverty, illiteracy, and lack of basic healthcare and amenities are perennial problems.
- The future needs are to ensure that the revised animal diseases legislation is approved and signed into law. Increased public awareness on good farm animal welfare practices on a species-by-species basis is necessary. It is also important to develop species-specific guidelines for good farm animal welfare.
- International NGOs are lacking in Nigeria, but their presence would help to implement government legislation, as well as to make welfare improvements through raising public awareness, educational campaigns and facilitating human behaviour changes.

8.6 Recommended Resources

- World Organisation for Animal Health website, https://www.oie.int/en/animal-welfare/animal-welfare-at-a-glance (accessed 8 April 2021).
- World Organisation for Animal Health Global Animal Welfare Strategy, https://www.oie.int/en/animal-welfare/oie-standards-and-international-trade (accessed 8 April 2021).
- World Organisation for Animal Health Terrestrial Animal Health Code, https://www.oie.int/standard-setting/terrestrial-code (accessed 8 April 2021).

References

Adesokan Lawal-Adebowale, O. (2020) Farm animals' health behaviours: An essential communicative signal for farmers' veterinary care and sustainable production. In: Abubakar, M. (ed.) *Livestock Health and Farming*. IntechOpen, London, doi:10.5772/intechopen.89738

Central Intelligence Agency (CIA) (2020) Africa: Nigeria – The World Factbook. Central Intelligence Agency. Available at: https://www.cia.gov/library/publications/the-world-factbook/geos/ni.html (accessed 21 August 2020).

Dixon, J., Gulliver, A., Gibbon, D. and Hall, M. (2001) *Farming Systems and Poverty: Improving Farmers' Livelihoods in a Changing World*. World Bank, Washington, DC.

Fayemi, P.O. and Muchenje, V. (2013) Maternal slaughter at abattoirs: History, causes, cases and the meat industry. *SpringerPlus* 2, 125. doi:10.1186/2193-1801-2-125

Proctor, H.S., Carder, G. and Cornish, A.R. (2013) Searching for animal sentience: A systematic review of the scientific literature. *Animals* 3, 882–906. doi:10.3390/ani3030882

Wilkins, D.B., Houseman, C., Allan, R., Appleby, M.C., Peeling, D. and Stevenson, P. (2005) Animal welfare: The role of non-governmental organisations. *OIE Revue Scientifique et Technique* 24, 625–638.

World Animal Protection (2020) Farm animal welfare. Available at: https://www.worldanimalprotection.org/our-work/animals-farming-supporting-70-billion-animals/farm-animal-welfare (accessed 28 June 2020).

World Organisation for Animal Health (OIE) (2019) Chapter 7.5 – Slaughter of Animals (OIE Terrestial Animal Health Code). Available at: https://www.oie.int/fileadmin/Home/eng/Health_standards/tahc/current/chapitre_aw_slaughter.pdf (accessed 28 June 2020).

9 Protecting Animals in India: A Government Perspective through History to the Present Day

Vijay Pal Singh[1] and Sujoy Khanna[2]
[1]*Council of Scientific and Industrial Research - Institute of Genomics and Integrative Biology, Delhi, India;* [2]*Lala Lajpat Rai University of Veterinary and Animal Sciences (LUVAS), Hisar, India*

> It shall be the fundamental duty of every citizen of India to protect and improve the natural environment including forests, lakes, rivers, and wildlife, and to have compassion for all living creatures. (The Indian Constitution 1976)

9.1 Introduction

Concern for animal welfare in India can be witnessed from as far back as 10,000 BCE. This chapter reminds us of the region's ancient views towards animals, following these through to the modern-day treatment of animals and animal welfare law. Beginning with some of the earliest records, archaeological excavations from as early as 2500 BCE, the pre-Vedic period, in the Indus valley show evidence of animal domestication for agricultural-draught and travel purposes (Bilimoria *et al.*, 2007). Although their use for work was the main reason for domestication, they were worshipped and treated as manifestations of higher-order beings. The 'Pashupathi seal' is a famous depiction of the early Hindu God called proto-Shiva ('father of animals'), who in this stone carving is surrounded by animals including elephants, tigers, water buffaloes and rhinoceros. This is regarded as evidence of the important role animals had in these civilizations.

The following Vedic period (1500–1000 BCE) saw many animals, such as cows, occupy a place of pride, worship, personification of motherhood, fertility and liberty (Bilimoria *et al.*, 2007). During this period, the Aryan people were known to have emphasized the protection of cows. During the latter part of this period, however, practices involving cow sacrifice gained pace to please the gods. Horses, ewes, goats, tortoises and other animals were also sacrificed with prayers in the belief of the different benefits this sacrifice would provide to people. However, the puranas (the ancient religious texts) of India advocated the co-existence of humans with nature. Lord Krishna expressed his love and devotion for cows rather than Lord Indra, a demi-god. He even advocated ensuring sufficient milk for calves before humans. These puranas prohibited the killing of animals for fun, or for food purposes, as this would upset the ecological balance of nature. Respect was bestowed upon old cows, retired war horses, and even diseased animals were provided with care and food. Severe punishments and heavy fines were prescribed for cruelty against animals. In 500 BCE, Buddha advocated against harm to all animals and birds, along with his preaching of non-violence towards humans.

During the Mauryan age (322–232 BCE), veterinary services were believed to be essential for animals and heavy fines were imposed for causing a bull to fight with another bull (Bilimoria et al., 2007). Protection of wildlife was ordered by Emperor Ashoka centuries before the concept of 'wild animal welfare' came into being. He erected the first known veterinary hospital in the world in 300 BCE (Somvanshi, 2006). There were widespread religious beliefs that all living beings, including humans and animals, go through a repeated cycle of reincarnation, with the souls of humans reincarnated as animals and vice versa. Animals were considered as reincarnated beings and perhaps of humans too.

Historical worship patterns in Indian society glorified many animals, in turn leading to their improved welfare. Many of these animals are still worshipped today. Elephants and monkeys are worshipped by large number of Indians as Lord Ganesha and Lord Hanuman, respectively. Rats, swans, bulls, lions and tigers are worshipped as the vehicles of Lord Ganesha, Brahma, Shiva and Goddess Durga, respectively. Jatayu, a wild bird, is worshipped for being a friend of Lord Rama. Above all of these, the sacred image of cows not only led to this animal being worshipped, but also to a movement called 'cow protection' in Hinduism, a major religion of India (Margul, 1968).

The ancient history of India had extraordinary contrasts in the treatment of animals, from sacrificing them for personal gains to worshipping them as immortals. Animals were reared by people not just to dominate over them, but to accommodate them as part of families. India has always been a multi-religious country, and different religions presented diverse views towards animal ethics. Jainism, Buddhism and, to a strong extent, Hinduism firmly believe that animals should not be used by humans as food (Szűcs et al., 2012), animal sacrifice should be abandoned and no injury should be wilfully made to any living being including animals. This makes India a society with a large section of the population vegetarian and with a love and compassion for animals.

Before independence, India had an active cow shelter (Dabra Pinjarapole) established since 1600, which inspired the creation of the Royal Society for Prevention of Cruelty to Animals (1824) in England. This was followed by the creation of the Calcutta Society for the Prevention of Cruelty to Animals (1861) by Colesworthey Grant, an English activist, to improve the conditions of draught animals. Since independence (1947), India has created extensive acts and laws to control the rearing, management, housing, transport, slaughter, killing for disease control and euthanasia of domestic animals. There are acts and laws for the welfare of domestic, wild, performing, laboratory and stray animals. For example, the Prevention of Cruelty to Animals (PCA) Act (1960) and the Wildlife Protection (WPA) Act (1972) were the landmark acts that laid a solid foundation of animal welfare laws and still determine the future course of animal welfare in India.

In 1986 computer-aided dissection was introduced for teaching to replace using animals. A series of steps were taken including the formation of the Animal Welfare Board of India (AWBI) and the Committee for the Purpose of Control and Supervision of Experiments on Animals (CPCSEA) to implement guidelines governing the use of animals in research. These brought India in line with other countries devoted to the welfare of animals.

In this chapter, we describe the welfare challenges and opportunities of modern-day India, with a particular focus on street animals and performing animals. We explore how ancient laws and religions have shaped today's society, the government and laws and how these are enforced, and the role of practitioners in India who want to make changes to benefit animal welfare (Fig. 9.1).

9.2 Work and Life as an Animal Welfare Practitioner

India has strong legislation to protect animals from abuse. But unlike humans, animals cannot raise voice for the rights they are entitled to, and are left with no option other than to suffer when these laws are not implemented. Animal welfare practitioners deal with animal cruelty, abuse and neglect, and improve their quality of life by raising their voice. In India, there are a wide range of welfare professionals, including degree holders in veterinary, animal or wildlife sciences, diploma holders in livestock handling, and trainees or interns with non-governmental organizations (NGOs), veterinary clinics, hospitals, cow shelters (Gaushalas, Fig. 9.2) and municipal animal birth control (ABC) programmes. There are also many welfare practitioners who do not have qualifications in animal welfare, but possess a love of animals and need to earn a livelihood. Although not professionally qualified, they tend to have a sound knowledge of animals because of long practical exposure in their respective fields, but generally their knowledge of acts, regulations and codes of practice for animal welfare is very limited.

The author Vijay has always been interested in animal welfare. He originally trained as a veterinarian and took a post in the government food safety department. An opportunity to attend an animal welfare course in the UK, run by animal welfare expert Professor Donald Broom, sparked his interest in animal welfare science. Vijay became involved with the International Society for Applied Ethology (ISAE), organizing the first ISAE animal behaviour and welfare science workshop in Delhi in 2018 and organizing the first international ISAE congress due to be held in Bangalore in 2020 but postponed by COVID-19. He is now a World Veterinary Association animal

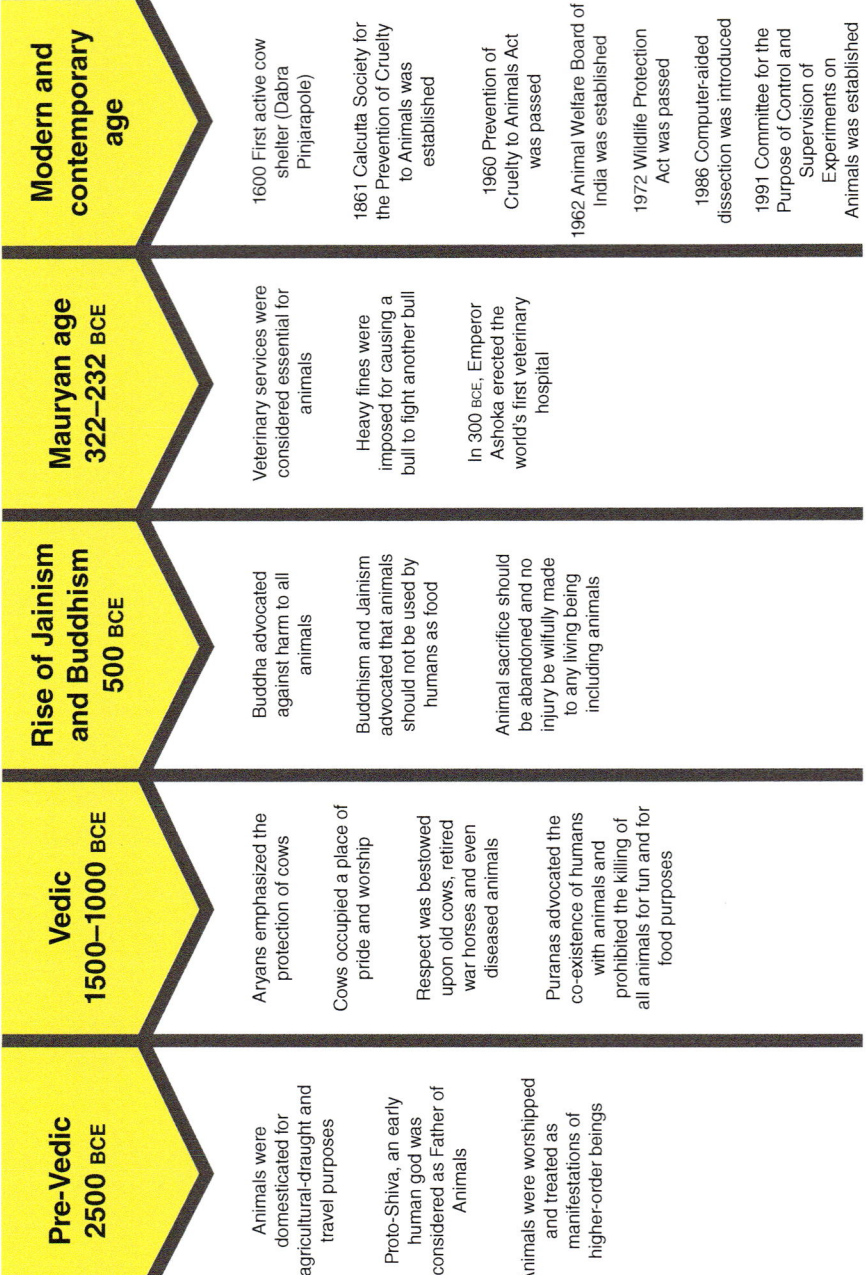

Fig. 9.1. A timeline of cultural attitudes to animals in India through the ages.

welfare representative for India. So while his day job focuses on other areas, he spends much of his own time on these projects he cares about.

The author Sujoy (Fig. 9.3) is a veterinarian with a PhD in livestock production management. He is a recipient of the INSPIRE fellowship from the

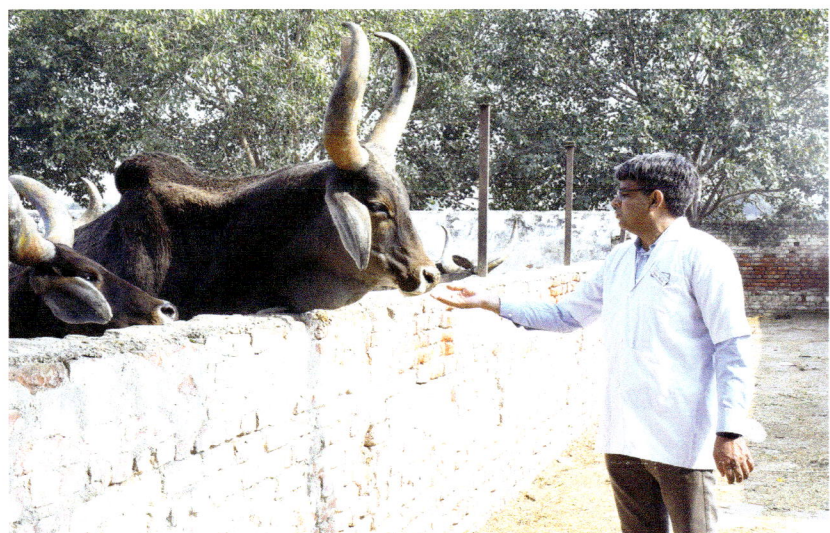

Fig. 9.2. Author Vijay treating stray cattle in a Gaushala (cow shelter).

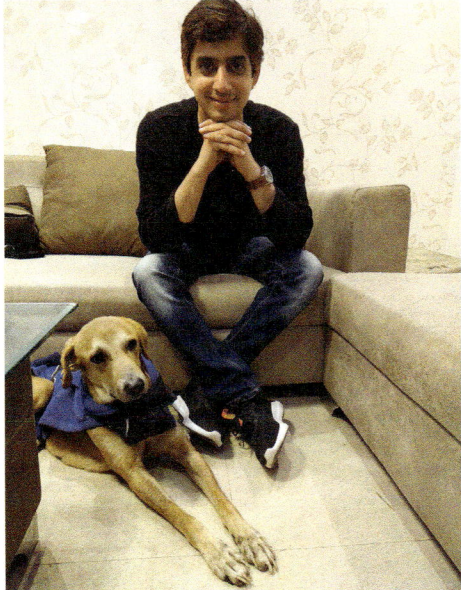

Fig. 9.3. Author Sujoy with his pet dog.

Ministry of Science and Technology, Government of India. He has worked as an assistant professor, Department of Livestock Production Management and as associate in charge, Disease Free Small Animal House, LUVAS. He wrote an influential book entitled *Gaushala* with Mrs Maneka Sanjay Gandhi, ex-cabinet minister and chair of the organization People for Animals aimed towards transforming the cattle shelters of India into loving homes for animals. While working on this book he aroused considerable interest in animal welfare activities and is currently working as an assistant professor and extension specialist looking after animal welfare activities, guiding animal owners on sustainable animal friendly management techniques and organizing vocational training, workshops and camps at a village grassroots level.

9.3 Improving Animal Welfare through Government in India

9.3.1 Street animals

9.3.1.1 Dogs

There are approximately 15.3 million stray dogs (Fig. 9.4) and 5.02 million stray cattle in India (Ministry of Fisheries, Animal Husbandry and Dairying, 2019). The vast majority of these animals were previously owned and cared for as companion, domestic and producing animals. The reason for their abandonment is reduced productivity in dairy and producing animals making them financially unviable, increasing age leading to development of various health issues in domestic and companion animals and, at times, development of issues like biting in companion animals. Following abandonment, these stray animals that were once cared for extensively by their owners are routinely subjected to ill-treatment and harassment. They have no means of feeding themselves and depend on begging from residential houses, offices, restaurants and roadside eateries (where they have easy access to food) for their survival. The population of stray animals has exponentially increased alongside high-density human population areas in cities. They are deprived of food and essential veterinary care, largely owing to a lack of measures to control their population. The main reasons for apparent free-roaming dogs (a portion do have owners or communities who care for them) (AWBI, 2011) are unregulated breeding, lack of responsible ownership, easy availability of food waste, exposed garbage and improper birth control measures. Abandoned pet dogs, if not rescued, continue to live on the streets and breed, adding to the existing street dog population, or get killed in road accidents.

There is a clear need to manage street dog populations efficiently to promote human and animal health and welfare, without causing animal suffering. Controlling dog populations brings down cases of dog bites and rabies. The mass killing of street dogs through various means, including

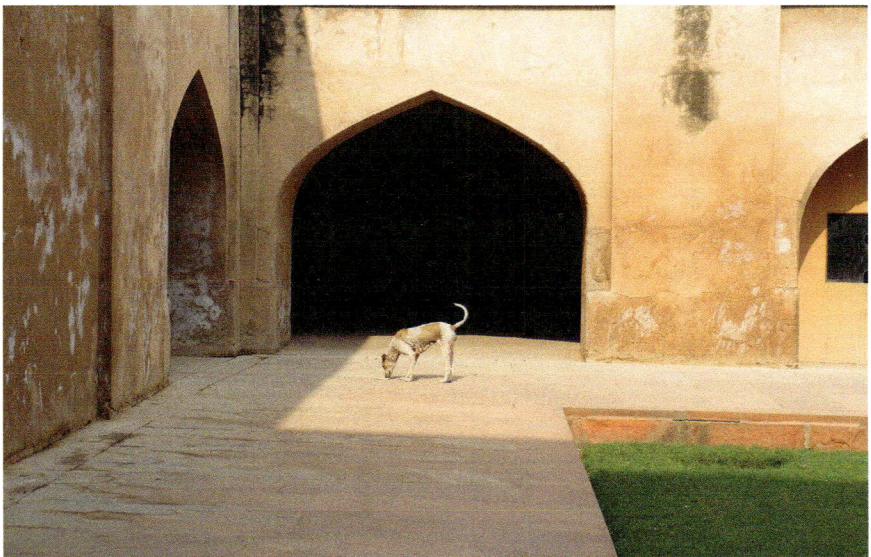

Fig. 9.4. A street dog at the Agra fort, India. (Photo courtesy of Rebecca Sommerville.)

electrocution, shooting and poisoning, was for a time seen as the only solution by authorities to control the street dog population and deaths caused by rabies. However, there is no correlation between the two (AWBI, 2011) and the unscientific killing, and the variable urban and rural conditions were not taken into account.

Street dogs that are removed or killed are easily replaced with new dogs from other territories, keeping the population growth steady. This was going on in India for more than 150 years until the Animal Birth Control (Dogs) Rules, 2001 were introduced, specifically forbidding the killing of street dogs and mandating birth control programmes, owing to pressure from animal welfare advocates. It was then that city municipal corporations and several NGOs in India began ABC programmes on a large scale as an alternative to killing stray dogs. A large number of street dogs in India are feral household dogs that are accepted by the community and belong to the neighbourhood. These animals are 'community owned' and people from the neighbourhood assume occasional responsibility for these dogs by feeding them, treating them when they are ill and getting them vaccinated; they typically don't allow birth control measures on the animal. By this, they intend to protect them from people they believe may harm them.

The trend for pedigree dogs has also increased among the Indian public. Many of these are genuine dog lovers, but there are people who acquire them on a whim, soon become tired of them and abandon them on the street. India should promote responsible dog ownership where owners have good knowledge of the behaviour and basic needs of dogs. It must also be ensured that dogs are properly vaccinated and treated against diseases. This way the abandonment issue of stray dogs could be resolved. City municipal corporations that are responsible for ABC programmes must be equipped with the human resources and infrastructure to handle it in a scientific way. Animal welfare organizations carrying out ABC programmes should follow humane catching and transportation procedures for stray dogs, along with identification methods and record keeping as prescribed by the guidelines of AWBI and the International Companion Animal Management (ICAM) coalition, discussed in Chapter 4. Anaesthetic protocols and pre- and post-operative care must also be followed by veterinary surgeons doing the ABC surgery to prevent harm being inadvertently caused.

Though the Animal Birth Control (Dogs) Rules were introduced in 2001, they are still not implemented with the seriousness they deserve. Funding for ABC programmes needs to be increased substantially for systematic implementation and enforcement across the country, in a planned phase-like manner. This would require better coordination between various Ministries including Urban Development, Health, Animal Husbandry and Environment, and other stakeholders. Preferential neutering should be carried out on street dogs for which complaints of habitual biting or unprovoked aggression are received to prevent these traits being passed on. Since pet dogs are potential stray animals, the focus should also be on regulating pet shops for homing or adoption of any pet animal that has not found a buyer. There has been a positive recent decline in the stray dog population (10.67%) as more middle-class urban families decide to keep stray dogs as pets, and also owing to the adoption of the ABC programme (Totton, 2009). Deployment of rigorous de-sexing programmes at animal welfare shelters and public veterinary hospitals, dispensaries and clinics would check the population of stray dogs. Furthermore, the general public, especially children, should be educated on how to approach and interact with dogs to prevent dog bites and rabies.

9.3.1.2 Cattle

The street cattle population of India mainly comprises cows – ironically because of religious sentiments and love towards these sentient beings preventing them from ending up in slaughterhouses. The buffaloes of the country are rarely found on the streets and end up in slaughterhouses after the end of their productive lifespan. For the street cattle, there are Gaushalas (Fig. 9.5), which are the institutions of India's great cultural heritage showing reverence and affection for animals, particularly cows, although some Gaushalas are also loving homes for buffaloes. The origin of these Gaushalas can be traced back to the Vedic period when social customs and rules laid great emphasis on protection, presentation and development of cows for the home and oxen for agricultural work. Protection and service of the cow was an article of

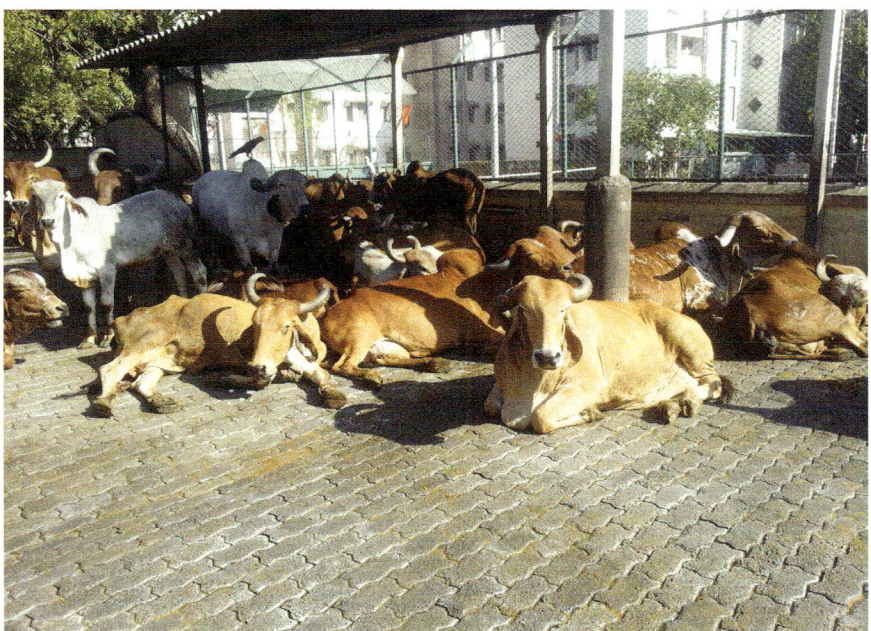

Fig. 9.5. Old, infertile or abandoned cattle in a Gaushala in Surat Pinjarapole, Gujarat State. (Photo courtesy of Arvind Sharma.)

faith and part of religion for Hindus. Even today, this faith is carried forward in Gaushalas – institutions where productivity and economics are not the driving force. These are set up side-by-side with modern dairy farms. The very fact that these Gaushalas have been concerned about cows in India for so long shows that cows to Indians are much more than a mere domestic animal. Since the purpose of Gaushalas is to provide a home to homeless cattle, it becomes incumbent upon the management of Gaushalas to ensure provision of the minimum basic needs of the housed cattle. However, large numbers of existing Gaushalas are overcrowded with poor feeding, housing and healthcare facilities. Therefore, their ability to meet minimum welfare standards leaves much to be desired.

The Gaushala in Fig. 9.5 is an almost century-old institution in the heart of a very busy city. It thrives on the philanthropy of local people and the thriving business community of the city. Cattle are fed concentrates along with fodder (dry and green). Overfeeding of concentrates by visitors, who visit this shelter for religious reasons as cows are considered sacred by the majority Hindu community in a country where cow slaughter is prohibited by law, leads to diarrhoea and other gastrointestinal problems. The flooring is interlocking concrete tiles that are easier for cleaning but may get slippery owing to continuous wear, leading to falls and injuries to the cattle. The cattle also sustain bruises and extensive wounds to their joints and extremities owing to regular contact with such surfaces.

With a human population of 1.37 billion and a stray animal population of 20 million in India (Ministry of Fisheries, Animal Husbandry and Dairying, 2019), for every stray animal there are more than six human beings. The human population of India can easily cater to their needs in theory. Yet one cannot be happy with the gigantic stray animal figures, given their poor state of being all over the country. Therefore, the need of the hour is to implement stray animal population control programmes, open more new modern animal shelters and Gaushalas, and upgrade the existing Gaushalas so that all free-roaming cattle are accommodated properly and their welfare can be ensured.

9.3.2 Performing animals

India has a long history of traditional animal performers called 'Madaris' or 'Kalandars'. These were the employed entertainers of the royal courts of kings, who used animals for performance long before welfare laws were made. With intensified raids against them for violation of the PCA Act, 1960 and the WPA Act, 1972 their numbers substantially reduced. Yet animals continue to be used for the purpose of entertainment in films, circuses or equine animal events to which the public are admitted. These animals are required to be registered in the Online System for Performing Animal Registration on the AWBI website and currently India has 200 performing animals.

> **Case Study 1: Jallikattu Bull Taming**
>
> Jallikattu is an ancient bull taming sporting event associated with the Pongal harvest festival. It is one of the most ancient living sports of Indian and Tamil history that is still widely prevalent. Jallikattu literally means grabbing a bag of coins tied to the horns of the bull (Kalaiyarasan, 2017). It was known as a sport where men displayed their bravery by overpowering a loose bull in the arena and tried to win the prize of coins tied to its horns. The bulls could be confronted by a single person or a group of people.
>
> Historically, chivalrous young men who were successful at Jallikattu were chosen by Tamil women to be their husbands. This sport was a way of expressing male prowess (Jayashree et al., 2019). Today, Jallikattu involves young men competing against the bulls and trying to hold onto the horns or embrace the hump to subdue a bull for a specified time within an enclosed arena. The organizers of this traditional sport, in order to incite ferocity in the bull and make the event more competitive and exciting, indulge in many malpractices, increasing the pain and distress of the already terrified animal. The bull's natural nervousness as a prey animal is exploited by the humans when they are released into a large and terrifying crowd. The bulls are deliberately made to feel afraid and out of fear they run away from the crowd. The bulls in the arena experience both fear and pain. Post-game examination of bulls reveals multiple cuts to the ears, and mutilation and dislocation of the tail bone.

Continued

Continued.

Jallikattu is argued to be a legitimate part of Tamil culture. It has been taking place for generations and the bulls are revered. Politics added fuel to the desire to retain the sport after it was banned by the Supreme Court of India in 2014 (Drennan, 2017). The Supreme Court verdict of the Jallikattu ban was based on the overwhelming evidence of abuse and cruelty demonstrated by the AWBI (Vignesh, 2018). Intense protests in favour of 'Jallikattu' and 'Tamil culture' broke out to reinstate the sport. Mass support grew to put pressure on the state government. They saw the ban as an attack on Tamil culture and pride, while those in favour of the ban were portrayed as anti-Tamil. The urban protest for a rural issue transcended the rural–urban divide of society. In a rare occurrence of collusion, both the State government and the central government flattened a court judgment, overruling the ban in 2017. The Tamil Nadu government released guidelines, some of which aimed towards improving the conditions of the Jallikattu bulls, such as ensuring that the inspection team of AWBI have a representative monitoring the event.

Culture is no excuse for cruelty. Such a practice is not worthy to be carried forward into the current century and undermines the bull's right to live and experience good welfare. Cultural and traditional relevance are being used as a shield to allow the practice. India has in the past successfully ended the age-old tradition of bear dancing (see Chapter 10). A sustainable solution can be created with participation of governments, communities and different stakeholders. Although the ban was short lived, it improved the morale of animal welfare stakeholders towards the ultimate goal of banning the exhibition and training of all performing animals. It will take time and collaboration to bring a change in the tradition, practice and perspective of people to end it. Only a complete ban can mean no more animal suffering.

How to Change the Behaviour of Owners of Captive Performing Elephants

The Indian elephant (*Elephas maximus*) is a unique example as it is the only wild animal in India that is protected under the WPA Act, 1972, yet is still used for entertainment purposes (Fig. 9.6). Close to 2500 elephants are kept in poor conditions in captivity. Elephants are very emotional, sentient and social intelligent beings, and health and behavioural clinical signs of suffering develop in performing elephants. The majority are registered with private owners, and the remainder with temples, zoos and circuses. Despite the WPA Act, 1972, an exception was created for captive elephants. Private owners are required to possess a certificate of ownership or make a declaration to the Chief Wildlife Warden or the authorized officer. Over the decades, this became an on-going mechanism to maintain private ownership of elephants and has been misused to capture new elephants from the wild.

Centuries-old practices are seen in some of the southern states of India, such as Kerala, where elephant rearing is considered part of their vibrant culture. In 2016, AWBI issued an advisory describing the cruelty endured by elephants when they are used for training and exhibition as well as forcing them to perform tricks that are unnatural to them. Taking a step forward, the environment ministry, in a draft notification in 2018, invited comments from various stakeholders within 30 days,

Continued

Continued.

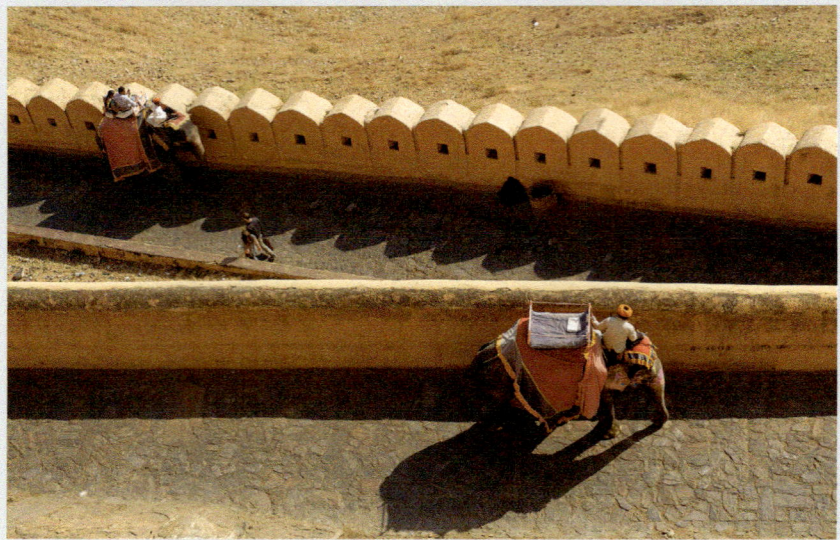

Fig. 9.6. Elephants working in tourism can experience many welfare challenges. These elephants are working at the city palace, Jaipur, India. (Photo courtesy of Rebecca Sommerville.)

after which the use of all animals including elephants for performances, exhibition at any circus or mobile entertainment facilities would be banned. After this, strict guidelines were put in place by the Ministry of Environment, Forests and Climate Change for enforcing animal welfare.

Recommendations for decision makers moving forward

- A ban on the use of elephants as performing animals would inch India closer to being the progressive compassionate nation that is embedded in its historical background.
- A clear-cut and comprehensive order for implementation of the acts and rules by central government would ensure better protection of the elephants in India.
- The Ministry of Environment, Forests and Climate Change should issue a central notification, with exercise of powers conferred to it by Section 22 of the PCA Act, 1960, to ban the training, exhibition and use of elephants for performances in India. A similar notification earlier banned bears, monkeys, tigers, panthers, lions and bulls from being exhibited or trained as performing animals, which has been effective. We see hardly any street or circus performances by these animals.
- The elephants in private ownership should be vigorously checked for violation of the statutory provisions of the PCA Act, 1960, Performing Animal Rules, 1973, the Performing Animals (Registration) Rules, 2001, WPA Act, 1972, Recognition of Zoo Rules, 2009, and the guidelines issued on care

Continued

Continued.

and management of captive elephants by the Central Zoo Authority (CZA) and Project Elephant Division. AWBI, being the prescribed authority, may advise for strict criteria or even stop registration of elephants for performance to reduce the number of elephants undergoing pain and suffering.

- Elephant ownership certificates are issued for a period of 5 years and should be renewed every 5 years. Illegal elephants without valid documents should be confiscated and arrangements should be made for their return to the wild or safe sanctuary.
- AWBI should take note of the deplorable conditions of elephants even after giving several chances to the circus operators and revoke and deregister the use of all elephants in circuses with immediate effect. Elephants abused in circuses should be seized and housed in elephant camps or rehabilitation centres with the help of Chief Wildlife Wardens. The complaints received by AWBI regarding the abuse of captive elephants have increased substantially, showing awareness of the general public towards the cause of elephants.
- If a blanket ban is not imposed, then agencies should stress measures like better training for mahouts (elephant handlers), serving more nutritious food to the animals, and improved veterinary care and housing facilities. For instance, according to the guidelines of CZA, an elephant should be provided with a large forested or vegetative environment, lakes and a water body, in addition to being housed in groups with a minimum space requirement of 1.2 acres per elephant.
- Indian people are increasingly becoming aware that elephants suffer in captivity and should not be kept in exploitative conditions. With the decline in number of circuses, it is clearly evident that educated and compassionate citizens of India have rejected circuses and even reduced their participation in elephant parades for entertainment.

9.4 Overcoming Challenges

The major problems (and the forces behind them) faced by animal welfare practitioners in their quest towards protecting and safeguarding animals have been identified. Within these problems lie opportunities for further improving the welfare state of animals. India was one of the first countries to enact a law on the subject of animal cruelty through the PCA Act, 1960. However, relatively weak penalties for violation in addition to an absence of proactive and pre-emptive measures for the prevention of animal cruelty prevent this legislation from being as successful as was intended. Animal welfare is very often considered synonymous with animal health in India, but animal welfare is more than that and requires special effort. Though the health condition of animals has improved owing to the concerted efforts of veterinarians and other animal welfare professionals, a lot is still to be achieved for the welfare state of animals.

Government agencies who formulate policies are entirely focused on the production outputs of animals. The animal welfare divisions of government are staffed by junior bureaucrats holding multiple charges to look after the administration, with little attention paid to the scientific aspect. Ethical angles to policies after proper scientific consideration should be embedded while policy making. The political class lack focused critical thinking on animal welfare, except for the welfare of cows. This prioritization of cow welfare in India, with steps that lack scientific evidence, negatively impacts the overall welfare of animals.

The animal welfare practitioners of India, such as the National Animal Welfare Advisory Committee, have a very limited role in drafting animal welfare laws. Lack of transparency, trust and openness in organizations (NGOs, institutes, etc.) that receive funds from the government or the public is a major driver for misutilization or underutilization of funds meant for the welfare of animals. This lack of transparency lowers the donors' trust and tarnishes the image of the organization. Thus, these organizations must be made to publish their reports.

Indian society has at many times shown a reluctance to deviate from cultural, social and religious practices as well as from the conventional understanding of the wellbeing of animals. This reluctance to change, which was recently evident in the case of the Jallikattu festival, hinders the ultimate aim of improving the wellbeing of animals.

9.5 Conclusions

After independence, India laid a good foundation of animal welfare by enacting the PCA Act in 1960 to prevent the infliction of unnecessary pain or suffering on animals. The WPA Act of 1972 is one of the strictest wildlife protection acts in the world. These acts have been utilized by AWBI, NGOs and other stakeholders to appeal to the government against acts committed towards animals that cause suffering. In the past few decades, animal welfare practitioners in India have witnessed some of the biggest triumphs over conventional outdated animal practices, such as the ban on exhibition and training of five species of performing animals (bears, monkeys, tigers, panthers and lions) (1998), the Animal Birth Control (Dogs) Rules (2001), the PCA (Pet Shop Rules) Rules (2018) and many more. The Ministry of Environment, Forests and Climate Change notification banned the use of bulls as performing animals (2011), thereby banning the Jallikattu bull taming event. Although the ban was short lived, it strengthened the morale of the animal welfare stakeholders towards attaining the ultimate goal of banning the exhibition and training of all performing animals.

In India, acts and rules based their recommendations for animal welfare on scientifically justified practices. There have been a few setbacks by the government, however, after recognizing the influence these acts and rules have on the cultural and religious practices of society. More research on anthropomorphism, to change the perception of people towards animal welfare, will further improve the implementation of these acts and rules. India looks committed to the development of even better science-based welfare standards, despite the complex interplay of factors such as socio-economic conditions, culture, religion and tradition.

Mahatma Gandhi once said, 'The greatness of a nation and its progress can be judged by the way its animals are treated'. India today is placed on the world map as a scientifically progressive country that cares for its animals. A widespread acceptance of animal protection as a serious social issue and the better role of different institutions and agencies in animal cruelty would make India revisit its history of protecting animals by reducing the vested economic interests of society. India has the historical roots, potential and will to lead the world towards improved animal welfare.

9.6 Recommended Resources

- Animal Welfare Board of India, http://awbi.in (accessed 9 April 2021).
- Animal Welfare Division (Ministry of Fisheries, Animal Husbandry and Dairying), https://dahd.nic.in (accessed 9 April 2021).
- The Bombay Society for the Prevention of Cruelty to Animals, https://bombayspca.org (accessed 9 April 2021).
- Department of Animal Husbandry and Dairying, Government of Haryana, http://pashudhanharyana.gov.in (accessed 9 April 2021).
- State Agriculture/Veterinary Universities (LUVAS, Hisar), https://www.luvas.edu.in (accessed 9 April 2021).
- Central Agriculture Universities (Central Agricultural University, Imphal), https://www.cau.ac.in (accessed 9 April 2021), Rani Lakshmi Bai Central Agricultural University, Jhansi, www.rlbcau.ac.in (accessed 9 April 2021), Dr Rajendra Prasad Central Agricultural University, Samastipur, https://www.rpcau.ac.in (accessed 9 April 2021).
- Krishi Vigyan Kendras, part of the National Agricultural Research System, https://kvk.icar.gov.in (accessed 9 April 2021).
- National Institute of Animal Welfare, http://moef.gov.in/wp-content/uploads/2017/10/Annexure-1.pdf (accessed 9 April 2021).
- Animal welfare organizations – People for Animals, https://www.peopleforanimalsindia.org (accessed 9 April 2021), World Animal Protection, https://www.worldanimalprotection.org (accessed 9 April 2021) and People for the Ethical Treatment of Animals, https://www.petaindia.com (accessed 9 April 2021).

References

Animal Welfare Board of India (AWBI) (2011) Revised module for street dog population management, rabies eradication, reducing man–dog conflict. Available at: www.awbi.org/awbi-pdf/SOP.pdf (accessed 8 December 2020).

Bilimoria, P., Prabhu, J. and Sharma, R. (2007) *Indian Ethics: Classical Traditions and Contemporary Challenges* (Vol. 1), 2nd edition. Routledge, New York.

Drennan, V.S. (2017) Jallikattu and the art of legal dodging. The Hindu Centre for Politics and Public Policy. Available at: (https://www.thehinducentre.com/the-arena/current-issues/article9502154.ece (accessed 23 June 2021).

Jayashree, B., Aram, A. and Ibrahim, Y. (2019) The voices of culture, conservation and the media event around bullfight 'Jallikattu' in Tamil Nadu, India. *Journal of Media and Communication Studies* 11(3), 20–30.

Kalaiyarasan, A. (2017) Politics of Jallikattu. *Economic and Political Weekly* 6, 10–13.

Margul, T. (1968) Present-day worship of the cow in India. *Numen International Review for the History of Religions* 15(1), 63–80.

Ministry of Fisheries, Animal Husbandry and Dairying (2019) 20th livestock census – 2019. All India report. Government of India, New Delhi.

Somvanshi, R. (2006) Veterinary medicine and animal keeping in ancient India. *Asian Agri-History* 10(2), 133–146.

Szűcs, E., Geers, R., Jezierski, T., Sossidou, E.N. and Broom, D.M. (2012) Animal welfare in different human cultures, traditions and religious faiths. *Asian-Australas Journal of Animal Science* 25(11), 1499–1506.

Totton, S. (2009) Stray dog population health and demographics in Jodhpur, India following a spay/neuter/rabies vaccination program. PhD thesis, the University of Guelph, Ontario, Canada.

Vignesh, S. (2018) Hugging the bull: Becoming-animal in Jallikattu. *Deleuze and Guattari Studies* 12(1), 126–146.

10 The Animals Powering the World: Promoting Working Animal Welfare in Resource-poor Contexts

Ashleigh F. Brown
International animal behaviour and welfare scientist

10.1 Introduction

There are an estimated 200–300 million animals working in the service of humans around the world (Chirgwin, 1996; World Animal Net, 2017; SPANA, 2020), supporting many millions of people and contributing valuably to society through creation of economic and social capital. Animals undertake a broad range of work types including military and police support (e.g. mounted police, army pack mules), medical assistance (e.g. guide dogs, medical detection dogs) and entertainment (e.g. marine mammal performances). However, the large majority of working animals are engaged in the 'three Ts' of transport, traction or tourism, which will be the focus of this chapter. Species undertaking transport and traction activities are predominantly bovids (oxen, buffalo, yaks, cows), equids (horses, donkeys, mules) and camelids (camels, llamas); whereas tourism involves a wide range of domestic and exotic species, including elephants, big cats, birds, primates, reptiles and bears (Moorhouse *et al.*, 2015; Tourism Concern, 2017). This chapter will explore the welfare challenges working animals face and how to ameliorate these through the application of animal welfare science and supporting others to develop this knowledge.

Working animals – defined here as those reared and kept primarily for the purposes of conducting physical activities directed by people – are predominantly distributed within low- and middle-income countries, where they undertake vital roles that support livelihoods of individuals, families and communities, and bolster local and national economies (Chirgwin, 1996; Mengjie and Yi, 1996; FAO, 2014; Alves, 2018). These animals offer an efficient and ecologically sustainable source of draught power when alternatives are unsuitable or unaffordable, facilitate independent entrepreneurship and alleviate the burden of domestic tasks, particularly for women and girls (Curran and Smith, 2005; Mburu *et al.*, 2012; Valette, 2014).

Working animals contribute to:

- *Direct income generation.* Either worked by their owners or loaned to other users, animals are used to provide chargeable services such as transportation of people or goods (including construction and extractive industries (Fig. 10.1); Dowson, 2015; Mitra and Valette, 2017), tourism experiences or participation in traditional ceremonies, thus enabling independent business and providing important services to wider communities.
- *Indirect income generation.* Animals can support opportunities for secondary income-generating activities; for example, carrying produce to markets for sale, conveying mobile shops, or transporting owners or users to workplaces.
- *Domestic and social support.* Animals transport domestic necessities such as water and firewood, and bring children to school, people to medical facilities and women to antenatal care (e.g. Blua, 2013; BBC, 2015). In addition to facilitating use of otherwise inaccessible services, animals reduce time and energy required for domestic tasks, enabling this to be redirected to alternative activities such as education, child-rearing, employment or political engagement (Valette, 2014).
- *Subsistence and food security.* Working animals provide agricultural draught power in locations where motorized farming machinery is unaffordable or unsuitable for the terrain, which is particularly important for small-scale farming and pastoralist communities (Chirgwin, 1996; Committee on World Food Security, 2019), and improve efficiency and scale of farming,

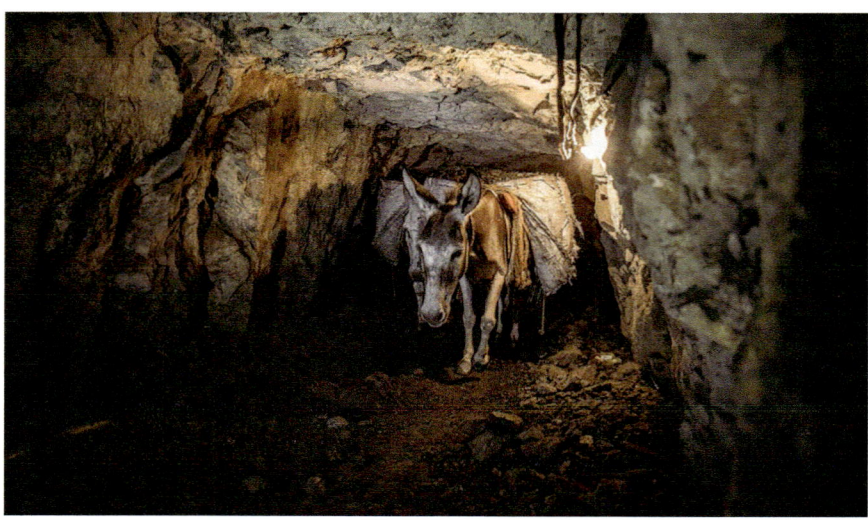

Fig. 10.1. A donkey toils in a dim and narrow mine shaft in Chakwal, Pakistan. (© Freya Dowson/Brooke.)

increasing food security (Mburu *et al.*, 2012). With an estimated 2.5 billion people dependent on agriculture for subsistence or livelihood (FAO, 2014), these animals offer a lifeline for many living in material poverty.

Through these activities, working animals contribute economic and social capital that can be leveraged and magnified through secondary benefits such as increasing financial stability and elevating social status. The working animal context thus represents an intersectionality between animal welfare and international development and, as long as there are working animals in resource-poor locations, animal welfare and human wellbeing will continue to be inextricably linked.

10.2 Work and Life as an Animal Welfare Practitioner

The author completed a Master of Science degree in applied animal behaviour and animal welfare, building on a background of practical work with horses and undergraduate studies in equine science. Appreciating the importance of educational, training and communication skills, she also gained professional qualifications in adult education and teaching English to speakers of other languages. In response to growing realization of the importance of effective governance in the non-governmental organization (NGO) sector, the author undertook a second Master's degree in international development management, and joined the board of trustees for two wildlife and conservation charities. Keen to support others' learning and development, she has also provided career mentoring to young people, academic supervision to animal welfare students, and has written research summaries for World Animal Protection's Global Animal Network.

Committed to working closely with animals, communities and international colleagues in the field, the author has practical experience with rescued 'dancing' sloth bears in India; tourism elephants in Thailand (Fig. 10.2); training horses in Scotland, Argentina and Canada; and has held scientific advisory positions at a leading working equine charity (Brooke) for more than a decade. Her professional interests include training others in animal welfare, behaviour and handling; developing welfare assessment methodologies; environmental enrichment and optimizing welfare in captivity; stereotypic and abnormal behaviour; mitigating animal welfare risk in projects and emergency response; and advising on equine-specific topics including farriery, harnessing and lorinery. Having worked or travelled in more than 75 countries to date, she learned the importance of cultural sensitivity, contextual adaptation and creation of in-country animal welfare expertise.

Reflecting on many years of practice with working animals internationally, five key areas of expertise emerged as important for operating effectively in this sector. These are based on the author's perceptions and learnings, and other practitioners may have alternatives to share, but

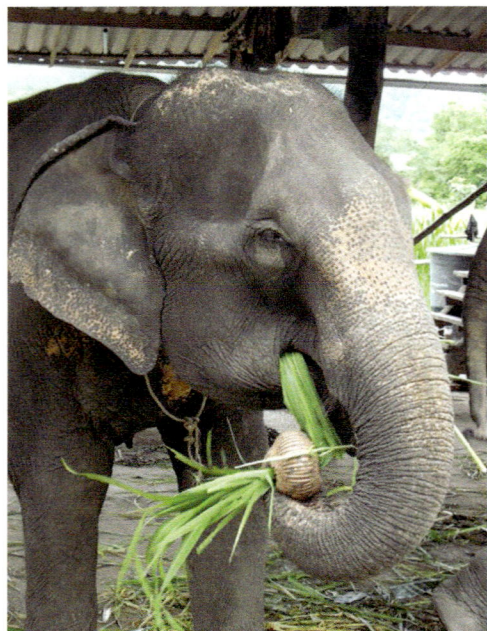

Fig. 10.2. Many Asian elephants who traditionally worked in logging and heavy goods transportation found alternative work in the tourism sector, presenting different welfare challenges. (Image: Ashleigh Brown.)

they should offer some guidance for current and aspiring animal welfare practitioners interested in working animals.

10.2.1 Animal welfare science

Knowledge of animal welfare concepts, ethics and science (as discussed in Chapter 1) is fundamental to underpin and inform practice, define objectives and requirements of interventions and justify their validity. Species-specific knowledge of physical and psychological requirements for good welfare is a prerequisite to designing activities that successfully meet those needs.

Animal welfare science is itself informed by ethology, the science of animal behaviour. Having an understanding of working species' behavioural norms enables consideration of ways in which natural behaviours may be thwarted or optimized in the working context; opportunities for positive welfare; and how instinctive responses influence human–animal interaction, safety and welfare. Appreciating the role of learning theory in relation to training, handling and instruction of animals during work is also important. Enhanced competence as a practitioner is derived from applying and embedding theoretical knowledge of ethological principles into practice in the field.

Since working animals are typically handled frequently (presenting both a welfare risk and positive welfare opportunity), the quality of the human–animal relationship is a major contributor to their daily and lifetime experience, and competence in animal handling is crucial for animal welfare practitioners to demonstrate good practice, train others, assist with challenging animals and maintain professional respect. Most working animal species are large and powerful, and the inability to handle them safely and humanely not only jeopardizes credibility with communities, but risks physical harm to animals and people. Practical 'hands-on' experience is essential to gaining skills and confidence in animal handling, which takes time, practice and patience. It is also important to acknowledge limitations and understand when to seek assistance from someone with greater capability. Individuals with reduced mobility or disability that inhibits directly handling animals should not feel excluded from pursuing work in this sector, as much valuable knowledge can be gained from closely observing animals' behaviour and interactions with each other and people.

An ability to apply scientific rigour to research, welfare assessment, monitoring and impact assessment processes has always been important in academia and research, but is increasingly valued and expected by donors in the NGO sector, who, quite rightly, seek evidence of impact and efficacy.

10.2.2   Contextual awareness

It is important for non-local practitioners to accept that without substantial lived experience in the operational environment it may not be possible to truly understand the daily realities for people who live and work there. However, willingness to learn about the society, gain exposure to the work context, and appreciate the challenges, motivations and barriers is a valuable prerequisite to operating effectively in a cultural context very different from one's own.

A fundamental error is attempting to treat variant contexts similarly, applying activities that have been successful elsewhere to a new location without adequately adapting. Apparent similarities on a superficial level can often mask important differences, and cultural nuances should not be overlooked. Culturally appropriate behaviour is important for nurturing a relationship of mutual respect, and as stakeholders typically engage with animal welfare practitioners and organizations voluntarily, maintaining these relationships is paramount to avoid causing disengagement or even offence. Understanding appropriate greetings, gender-specific interactions, and clothing and hairstyles, among others, supports this.

Awareness of how personal characteristics such as gender, age, ethnicity, nationality, language/dialect, socioeconomic background, education, mannerisms, marital status, etc. may be perceived and affect others' responses, and fostering a mindset of critical cultural awareness, support constructive collaboration. Being an 'outsider' can be both a hindrance and a help. For example, attracting a lot of attention can present an opportunity to demonstrate kindness towards animals to many interested onlookers, but can also add pressure when 200 people are watching every move! Even if working in one's home country or sharing characteristics with local people, being cognisant of how perceived 'otherness' may manifest is important, especially if conducting qualitative or social research when findings are influenced by a researchers' demographic (Brink, 1993; Frost *et al.*, 2010). At times it may be preferable for someone else to undertake certain activities, and having the personal capacity to reflect and acknowledge this – without prejudice or offence – is valuable and can be an important safety consideration. Externality and 'otherness' is not a barrier to successful collaboration – and in fact can be an asset – but lacking critical cultural awareness of fundamental differences in worldviews, inequality and positions of privilege may be (Lebedko, 2013; Christopher *et al.*, 2014).

10.2.3 Human behaviour

Working animals are owned by people, and are often their legal property without recognized independent rights (Animal Protection Index, 2020). Therefore, in order to influence what happens to these animals it is necessary to work directly with people. Understanding the rationale behind stakeholders' practices is a prerequisite to influencing them, and animal welfare practitioners can benefit greatly from gaining knowledge in human behaviour and psychology, and developing skills in engagement and facilitation (see Chapter 3). It is also important to collaborate with and learn from experts in social work, community engagement and advocacy, who can be valuable allies in stimulating positive behavioural change (see Chapter 4).

10.2.4 Development practice

Given the global distribution of working animals in resource-poor contexts, there are often socioeconomic needs in addition to animal welfare needs, and working in this sector in practice means operating at the intersection of animal welfare and international development. Accordingly, knowledge of the history, politics, socioeconomic and development landscape of the country/region is an important lens through which to consider how animal welfare initiatives may complement development or humanitarian activities.

This intersectionality brings both opportunities and risks: opportunities for partnership and collaboration on interconnected issues, but risks of competing for resources and influence, of spreading conflicting messages or encountering 'engagement fatigue' by stakeholders being targeted by multiple actors. For example, animal-owning communities may be simultaneously targeted by initiatives around education, public health, micro-finance and female empowerment in addition to animal welfare, resulting in multiple requests from various practitioners pursuing differentiated agendas. This reiterates the importance of contextual awareness, and also of participatory design of activities in conjunction with communities (Burkey, 1992; Chambers, 1994; Colom, 2013) (see Chapters 2, 3 and 4).

10.2.5 Training and mentoring

Training others is crucial, both to magnify impact on animal welfare through cascading learning to people who can potentially influence many more (scale), and to create sustainable action that does not stop when the original practitioners depart or the project ends (longevity).

It is not essential to have academic qualifications to be a great teacher, and some of the best have no formal teacher training (or little formal education at all) but are excellent natural communicators. For example, the author has a colleague in Brooke India who became a master trainer in animal welfare and handling after initially being employed as a driver, as his talents were duly recognized. Conversely, sometimes highly qualified individuals demonstrate poor ability to connect, inspire and communicate in practice, and it should not be assumed that subject matter expertise implies the ability to transfer that knowledge effectively (as discussed in Chapter 3). Educating others is an important responsibility – with scope to disseminate poor practice as well as good – and warrants attention alongside the subject matter being taught.

10.3 Improving Animal Welfare as an NGO

10.3.1 Appraising welfare

Understanding the current and potential welfare status of working animals is the logical starting point for developing activities aimed at improving it. One way of approaching this task is to consider the process according to the following three levels of welfare appraisal (Table 10.1). Through proactively seeking information at each of these levels it is possible to build an understanding of welfare needs, constraints and opportunities, and develop a strategy for improvement in conjunction with relevant stakeholders.

10.3.2 Welfare problems

Appraising welfare should guide practitioners towards identification and prioritization of issues to be addressed, which will vary between working animal species and contexts. Working animals are susceptible to many of the same welfare challenges as other animal groups (e.g. infectious disease, parasitism,

Table 10.1. Levels of welfare appraisal.

Level	Key question	Practitioner notes
1: Animal	What is the animal telling us?	'Ask the animals' using animal-based welfare indicators. Various welfare assessment methods, many of which can be adapted for working animal species, are documented in the literature (e.g. Pritchard et al., 2005; Wemelsfelder and Mullan, 2014; CORDIS, 2015; Sommerville et al., 2018) Group-level welfare assessment methodologies will not reflect the inter-animal variation common among working animals, who are often worked, handled and trained individually, and vary in age, owner/user, history, health, etc. Assessing welfare at single-animal level is likely to be more informative and capture individual differences Many welfare assessment protocols provide a 'snapshot in time', and may not reveal all prior experiences or cumulative welfare issues. Consider exploring historical factors such as early rearing conditions, weaning practice, initial training for work, transportation, previous ownership and work types in addition to current status
2: Working and living environment	What factors are directly impacting the animal's welfare?	Consider how conditions differ between work and home, climate seasonality and periodic changes in husbandry and work (e.g. tourist season) Observe work and home environments and explore husbandry practices Owners/users can often explain reasons for positive or negative welfare factors, beliefs about animal management, resource constraints and root causes of welfare problems
3: External context	What factors are indirectly impacting the animal and owner/user?	Factors beyond direct control of owners/users include the animal healthcare infrastructure, policy environment and working regulations Explore the role of socio-cultural aspects such as gender roles, religion, security/conflict and education

accidental injury), but additionally face some that are particular to the working context, examples of which are presented in Fig. 10.3.

10.4 Overcoming Challenges

It is important to avoid presumptions about barriers or solutions to improving animal welfare without adequate situational analysis with local stakeholders. However, there are some common barriers which often apply in working animal contexts that are useful to explore. These are described in the following box.

HUMAN–ANIMAL INTERACTION

Beating, violent training and aggressive verbal interaction can cause fear, distress, injury, pain, negative anticipation and learned helplessness. Positive bonds with humans can be a source of stimulation, enrichment or comfort.

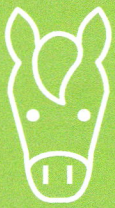

HARNESSING & EQUIPMENT

Pressure and abrasion create discomfort, pain, skin lesions and musculoskeletal problems. Comfortable and effective harness improves work efficiency, productivity, safety and reduces wasteful energy expenditure.

ACCOMMODATION & RESTRAINT

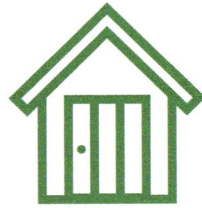

Isolation inhibits natural behaviour, and tethering can create injury and discomfort. Comfortable accommodation allows rest, protection, behavioural expression and monitoring of welfare.

Fig. 10.3. Examples of common welfare issues for working animals.

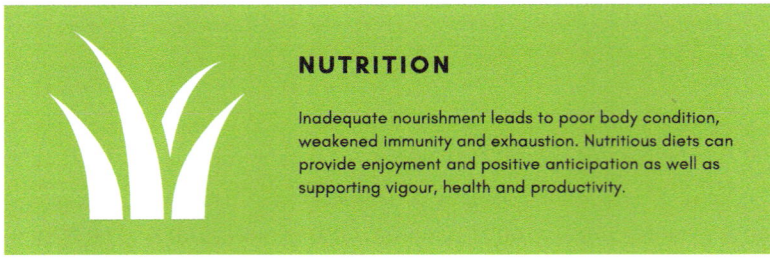

NUTRITION

Inadequate nourishment leads to poor body condition, weakened immunity and exhaustion. Nutritious diets can provide enjoyment and positive anticipation as well as supporting vigour, health and productivity.

WORKLOAD

Excessive physical demands cause exhaustion, poor body condition, tripping and risk of goading. Pleasant experiences between work (e.g. play, bathing) can offer respite and enrichment.

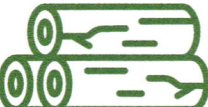

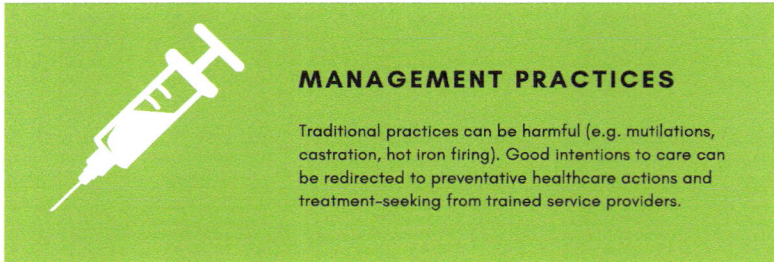

MANAGEMENT PRACTICES

Traditional practices can be harmful (e.g. mutilations, castration, hot iron firing). Good intentions to care can be redirected to preventative healthcare actions and treatment-seeking from trained service providers.

FEET & LIMBS

Lameness and joint abnormalities cause discomfort, pain, accidents and risk of goading. Pain-free walking can improve welfare with every step, increase productivity and support behavioural expression.

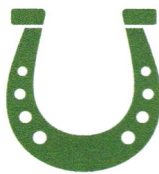

Fig. 10.3. Continued.

Addressing Barriers to Human Behaviour Change

1. Increase animal welfare knowledge

In many countries where working animals are prevalent there is little opportunity to formally learn about animal welfare, behaviour or ethics. There may not be widespread appreciation of animal sentience and suffering, nor even a word equivalent to 'welfare' in many dialects (FAO, 2014). There may be no examples of 'normal' or 'good welfare' in the animal population. This can manifest in poor

Continued

Continued.

treatment and a permissive social licence, meaning that violence or neglect towards animals is unchallenged. Solutions are to raise awareness of animal sentience, welfare and needs through educational initiatives in an appropriate format to targeted peoples' demographics.

2. Address financial pressures

People using animals for income are often under great pressure to increase the workload (e.g. size of load, quantity of trips, number of customers, speed of travel) to increase earnings, which predisposes to overloading, insufficient rest and goading. Owners or users may have very limited capacity to pay for adequate nutrition, healthcare and equipment. Ending financial poverty is multifactorial and requires engagement with livelihoods and development stakeholders. Many welfare improvements need not cost money – for example, removing harness during breaks, cleaning eyes, using humane training methods and finding shade – and practitioners should always identify these affordable, locally replicable solutions with owners and users.

3. Consider tradition and attitude

Harmful traditional practices (such as applying engine oil to wounds, violent training techniques or hot iron firing of skin) occur in many working animal contexts, sometimes perpetuated through myths and misunderstanding, and can be resistant to change as 'that's how it's always been'. Solutions involve first understanding the rationale behind the practice, then articulating what is problematic for the animal and owner (e.g. paying for something that actually harms the animal and hinders productivity), identifying acceptable alternatives and demonstrating their success. Engagement with children and young people is also important for influencing future practice (Arbour et al., 2009; Hawkins et al., 2017).

4. Address low status and recognition

Despite their valuable contribution, working animals are often perceived as low status, and may not receive essential care, veterinary treatment or protective policy (Swai and Bwanga, 2008; FAO, 2014). The low status and recognition of working animals is exacerbated because those in positions of influence often come from very different socioeconomic backgrounds from people who depend upon working animals, who are more likely to be living in rural, migrant or marginalized communities, and facing material poverty, financial instability and food insecurity. Quantifying the contributions of working animals and raising awareness of their value among stakeholders at both field and governance levels is important.

5. Foster engagement and participation

Active participation by owners and users in welfare-focused activities is integral to achieving sustainable improvement in practice, and constructive engagement between practitioners and communities is therefore crucial. Learning from community engagement and participatory practice within the (typically better-funded) fields of human healthcare, education and civil rights, enables practitioners to employ similar techniques for animal welfare improvement (Swann, 2006; van Dijk et al., 2011). Engagement and participatory techniques should be imple-

Continued

Continued.

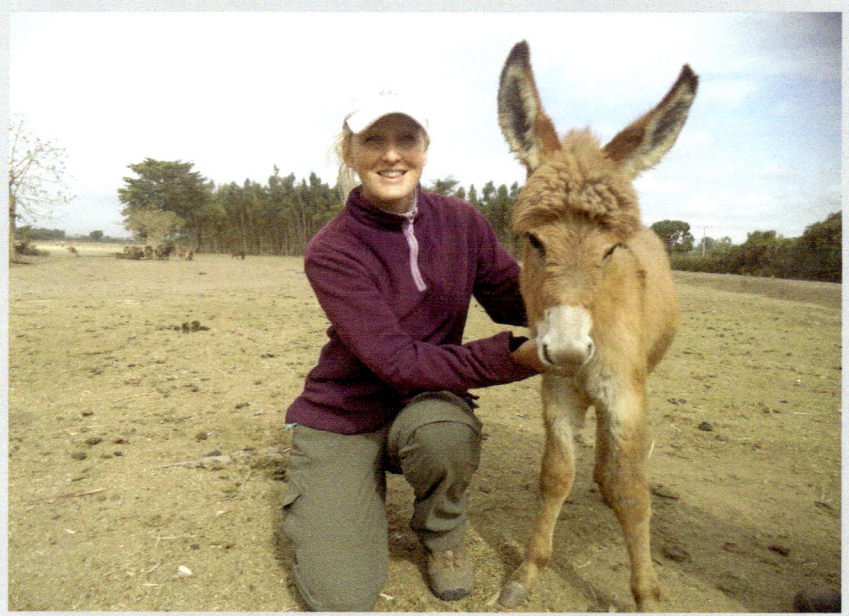

Fig. 10.4. Author Ashleigh spending a happy moment with a young foal in rural Ethiopia. Demonstrating positive interaction with working animals sets a good example to onlookers. (Image: Ashleigh Brown.)

mented reflectively and reflexively, critically evaluating efficacy and adapting to the context as required (see Chapter 4).

6. Provide alternatives to poor practice

Harmful traditional practices can be deeply entrenched and challenging to address, but opportunity for change can be presented through alternative practices that align with owners' or users' underlying motivations; for example, evidence-based veterinary treatment to counteract harmful traditional practice, or alternative livelihoods that do not require animal exploitation (see Case Study 1, this Chapter). A powerful motivator for change occurs when human benefit can result from animal welfare improvement, which is often the case with working animals since their productivity and longevity relates to their health and welfare status.

7. Enable in-country expertise

Development of in-country expertise is vital for long-term change and an attitudinal shift towards recognition of working animal welfare as a valid concern and respected discipline. Solutions should increase capacity at both local (field-based training of owners/users, animal health and welfare practitioners) and national levels (advocacy with policy makers, academics and educators), and supporting

Continued

Continued.

professional development of local practitioners should be prioritized over one-off interventions or sporadic activities run by external actors, such as NGOs.

8. Identify the change-makers and form alliances

Building relationships with the natural and unnatural allies is key. These may be high-status individuals such as religious leaders, tribal elders, government officials; or local community champions who can model good practice and encourage peers in positive change. Organizations or institutions with the power to influence and educate, such as media outlets and training facilities, are also important instruments for catalysing change. For animals working in tourism, the most influential stakeholders are often the tourists themselves who wield considerable consumer power, and the associated tour guides, agencies and regulatory bodies (e.g. ABTA, 2013).

9. Model positive behaviour

Positive influences in the field can result from animal welfare practitioners' behaviour towards animals when off duty. Practitioners should be mindful of which animals they notice, interacting positively with them, making ethical food choices and demonstrating compassion for all animals (Fig. 10.4). Interacting with working animals often requires operating in unpleasant or polluted surroundings (e.g. rubbish dumps, brick kilns), inhospitable terrain (e.g. deserts, mountains) or unsafe locations (e.g. crime-ridden or conflict-prone areas). Willingness to be immersed in these living and working conditions is important. It is not always possible to walk in others' shoes, but effort should be made to at least walk alongside them.

Case Study 1: Rescuing India's Dancing Bears

Despite being declared illegal since 1972, the traditional activity of 'bear dancing' had persisted among nomadic Kalandar people into the 21st century in India. Poaching of wild bear cubs had been encouraged within some tribes in the past, and these captured bears suffered severely owing to violence, inadequate nutrition, unsuitable living conditions, disease and being forced through painful methods to 'perform' publicly for payment. Successful interventions by Wildlife SOS and partners offered rescued bears comfortable retirement at their sanctuaries (Fig. 10.5), which drastically improved welfare in the short term; and these interventions were instrumental in reducing the practice throughout India and ultimately bringing it to an end in 2009 (International Animal Rescue, 2009; Schaul, 2012; Wildlife SOS, 2019), thus creating significant long-term change and preventing future suffering.

These outcomes were achieved through a combination of:

- effective collaboration between Wildlife SOS and the Indian government, state forest departments, law enforcement authorities and the Kalandar people (Schaul, 2012);
- consideration of future prevention in addition to addressing current animal suffering;
- strong understanding of relevant cultural and broader contextual factors;
- engagement with social issues (beyond animal protection alone); and

Continued

Case Study 1: Continued.

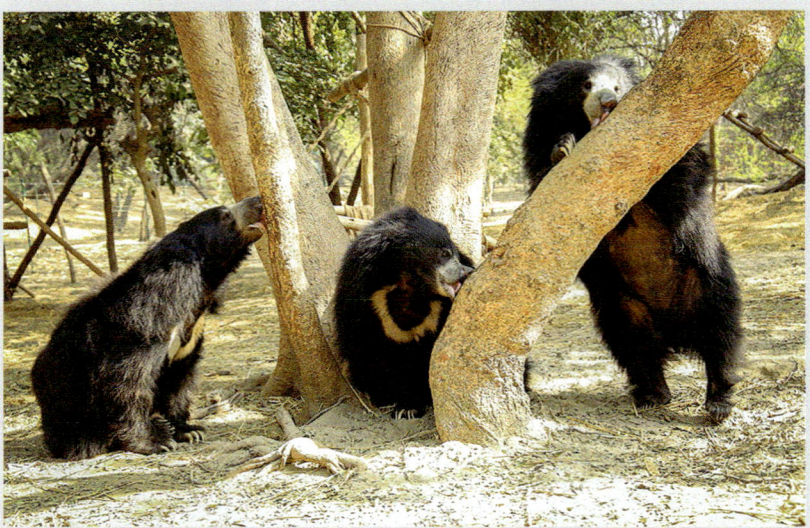

Fig. 10.5. Rescued sloth bears enjoy a safe and happy life in an enriched environment at Agra Bear Rescue Centre, India. (© Wildlife SOS.)

- species-specific welfare and behaviour knowledge to meet bears' needs in captivity.

Practitioners at Wildlife SOS understood that simply confiscating bears (which was legally plausible) would induce more poaching, because perpetrators would replace them in order to continue earning. To prevent this, bear owners were supported to establish alternative livelihoods, by providing seed funding and training to start small businesses such as craft making or food selling, thus removing reliance on bears (or other animals) (Schaul, 2012; *Deccan Chronicle*, 2018). This support was coupled with the potential for legal enforcement should reoffending occur, and perpetrators formally pledged never to remove another animal from the wild. Partnership with government and police gave credence and gravitas to these agreements; and partnership with perpetrators themselves was integral to establish trust, influence attitudes and create sustainable change. Some Kalandar people were even employed to care for rescued animals, having reformed their views on animal welfare and conservation (Ghai, 2014; K. Satyanarayan, 2008, pers. comm.).

This success story illustrates the importance of considering both short- and long-term animal welfare outcomes when planning welfare improvement and implementing solutions through fostering engagement with the key stakeholders and influencing behaviour change, forming strategic alliances and providing alternatives to poor practice that reflect the causative factors beyond animal welfare alone.

10.4.1 Outcome

Solutions for improving working animal welfare ultimately comprise two scenarios: changing conditions to enable acceptable welfare standards; or removing the need for the work (either to be done at all or to involve animals). There are some environments in which it may never be feasible to provide working animals a good quality of life (e.g. captive wildlife, extremely arduous work), and efforts should be directed towards reducing animal usage through abolition or mechanization and exploring alternative livelihoods for owners and users, in conjunction with ameliorating current suffering.

10.5 Conclusions

The future for working animal welfare will benefit from efforts to progress in the following areas:

- *Recognition of working animals' value.* The emergence of the One Welfare agenda has highlighted ways in which humans, animals and the environment are intertwined (Garcia Pinillos *et al.*, 2016), and the relevance of working animals – who interact so frequently with people and support livelihoods, food security and consequently impact human wellbeing – is evident. Greater research into working animal welfare, in terms of contextually feasible improvements and quantifying their socioeconomic contributions, may increase motivation to rectify welfare problems and improve associated support to the communities dependent upon them.
- *Reduced dependency on external intervention.* Formal education on (working) animal welfare and related topics is inaccessible to a global majority, and those with this privilege should consider how to support other current or aspiring practitioners' professional development in locations where it is needed most. Incorporating animal welfare content in educational curricula (including veterinary, agricultural engineering, animal sciences, economics, development and tourism sectors) would be a valuable step forward (de Boo and Knight, 2005; Allen *et al.*, 2017).
- *Preparedness for future challenges.* As a consequence of climate change coupled with a continually rising human population and associated land pressures, extreme weather phenomena, natural disasters, food security, water scarcity and interconnected conflicts are likely to increase (Reuveny, 2007; Werrell and Femia, 2018) and with them potentially the role of working animals. For example, rising oil prices previously resulted in increased utilization of animal traction (FAO, 2014); return of economic migrants to rural homelands during the COVID-19 pandemic resulted in uptake of animal-powered agriculture in Afghanistan (H. Nessar, 2020,

pers. comm.); and working animals have transported people fleeing conflict to refugee camps in Sudan (Pollock, 2018). Consequently it will become increasingly important to protect working animals and their supportive roles in communities in relation to prospective social and natural challenges.

Progress in each area will be enhanced through better integrating working animal welfare with other relevant fields, notably the international development sector and associated areas of education, healthcare, tourism and environment. It is both a tentative prediction and a heartfelt hope for the future that working animals receive greater attention from international and intersectional actors.

They are, after all, the animals powering the world.

10.6 Recommended Resources

- Animals Asia, https://www.animalsasia.org (accessed 9 April 2021).
- Born Free Foundation, https://www.bornfree.org.uk (accessed 9 April 2021).
- Brooke, https://www.thebrooke.org (accessed 9 April 2021).
- Donkey Sanctuary, https://www.thedonkeysanctuary.org.uk (accessed 9 April 2021).
- Gambia Horse and Donkey Trust, http://gambiahorseanddonkey.org.uk (accessed 9 April 2021).
- Humane Society International, https://www.hsi.org (accessed 9 April 2021).
- International Animal Rescue, https://www.internationalanimalrescue.org (accessed 9 April 2021).
- International Fund for Animal Welfare, https://www.ifaw.org (accessed 9 April 2021).
- People for the Ethical Treatment of Animals, https://www.peta.org (accessed 9 April 2021).
- The Society for the Protection of Animals Abroad, https://spana.org (accessed 9 April 2021).
- Tourism Concern, https://www.tourismconcern.org.uk (accessed 9 April 2021).
- Whale and Dolphin Conservation, https://uk.whales.org (accessed 9 April 2021).
- Wildlife SOS, https://wildlifesos.org (accessed 9 April 2021).
- Wild Welfare, https://wildwelfare.org (accessed 9 April 2021).
- World Animal Net, https://worldanimal.net (accessed 9 April 2021).
- World Animal Protection, https://www.worldanimalprotection.org (accessed 9 April 2021).
- World Horse Welfare, https://www.worldhorsewelfare.org (accessed 9 April 2021).

Acknowledgements

The author would like to thank all the educators, colleagues, communities and friends around the world who have taught her so much about theory and practice of improving working animal welfare. And, of course, the animals – the horses, bears, elephants, donkeys, camels and mischievous mules whose fortitude, patience and incredible good-heartedness in spite of their suffering at the hands of humans continually inspire and motivate.

Thank you to Jenni Nellist for review of this chapter and Rebecca Sommerville for chapter edits and infographic production.

References

ABTA (2013) Global welfare guidance for animals in tourism. The Travel Association. Available at: https://www.abta.com/sites/default/files/media/document/uploads/Global%20Welfare%20Guidance%20for%20Animals%20in%20Tourism%202019%20version.pdf (accessed 9 April 2021).

Allen, D., Hughes, C., Williams, R. and Bowles, D. (2017) Animal welfare in the national curriculum. Royal Society for the Prevention of Cruelty to Animals. Available at: https://politicalanimal.org.uk/wp-content/uploads/2017/06/AnimalWelfareintheCurriculum.pdf (accessed 9 April 2021).

Alves, R.R.N. (2018) The ethnozoological role of working animals in traction and transport. In: Alves, R.R.N. and Albuquerque, U.P. (eds) *Ethnozoology*. Academic Press, Cambridge, Massachusetts, pp. 339–349. https://doi.org/10.1016/B978-0-12-809913-1.00018-1

Animal Protection Index (2020) World animal protection. Available at: https://api.worldanimalprotection.org/about (accessed 9 April 2021).

Arbour, R., Signal, T. and Taylor, N. (2009) Teaching kindness: The promise of humane education. *Society and Animals* 17, 136–148. doi:10.1163/156853009X418073

BBC (2015) 'Donkey ambulance' saddles developed in Wales helping mothers. British Broadcasting Corporation. Available at: https://www.bbc.co.uk/news/uk-wales-north-west-wales-35151804 (accessed 9 April 2021).

Blua, A. (2013) 'Donkey ambulance' rides to the rescue of Afghan women in labor. Radio Free Europe/Radio Liberty. Available at: https://www.rferl.org/a/afghanistan-donkey-ambulance-maternity-saddle/25120705.html (accessed 9 April 2021).

Brink, H.I.L. (1993) Validity and reliability in qualitative research. *Curationis* 16(2), 35–38.

Burkey, S. (1992) *People First: A Guide to Self-Reliant, Participatory Rural Development*. Zed Books, London.

Chambers, R. (1994) Paradigm shifts and the practice of participatory research and development. Working paper 2. Institute of Development Studies, Brighton, UK. Available at: https://opendocs.ids.ac.uk/opendocs/bitstream/handle/20.500.12413/3712/WP2.pdf?seq (accessed 9 April 2021).

Chirgwin, J.C. (1996) Multipurpose use of animals. *World Animal Review* 86, 1996/1. FAO, Rome. Available at: www.fao.org/3/w0613t/w0613T01.htm#multipurpose%20use%20of%20animals (accessed 9 April 2021).

Christopher, J.C., Wendt, D.C., Marecek, J. and Goodman, D.M. (2014) Critical cultural awareness: Contributions to a globalizing psychology. *American Psychologist* 69(7), 645–655. https://doi.org/10.1037/a0036851

Colom, A. (2013) How to…avoid pitfalls in participatory development. *The Guardian*. Available at: https://www.theguardian.com/global-development-professionals-network/2013/apr/04/how-to-design-participatory-projects (accessed 9 April 2021).

Committee on World Food Security (2019) SE133: Pastoral mobility and working animal welfare in a changing landscape: Why policies should support adaptive initiatives to facilitate mobility, resource access and animal welfare. Available at: https://demo-sdg2.nuvole.org/news/committee-world-food-security-cfs-14-18-october-2019 (accessed 9 April 2021).

CORDIS (2015) Development, integration and dissemination of animal-based welfare indicators, including pain, in commercially important husbandry species, with special emphasis on small ruminants, equidae & turkeys. European Commission, Brussels. Available at: https://cordis.europa.eu/project/id/266213/reporting (accessed 9 April 2021).

Curran, M.M. and Smith, D.G. (2005) The impact of donkey ownership on the livelihoods of female peri-urban dwellers in Ethiopia. *Tropical Animal Health and Production* 37, 67–86. https://doi.org/10.1007/s11250-005-9009-y

de Boo, J. and Knight, A. (2005) 'Concepts in animal welfare': A syllabus in animal welfare science and ethics for veterinary schools. *Journal of Veterinary Medical Education* 32(4), 451–453. https://doi.org/10.3138/jvme.32.4.451

Deccan Chronicle (2018) Nine years of keeping sloth bears off the streets. Available at: https://www.deccanchronicle.com/nation/current-affairs/191218/nine-years-of-keeping-sloth-bears-off-the-streets.html (accessed 9 April 2021).

Dowson, F. (2015) Working donkeys and horses from around the world – in pictures. *The Guardian*. Available at: https://www.theguardian.com/global-development-professionals-network/gallery/2015/dec/22/working-donkeys-and-horses-from-around-the-world-in-pictures (accessed 9 April 2021).

Food and Agriculture Organization of the United Nations (FAO) (2014) The role, impact and welfare of working (traction and transport) animals. Animal Production and Health Report No. 5. FAO, Rome. www.fao.org/3/i3381e/i3381e.pdf (accessed 9 April 2021).

Frost, N., Nolas, S.M., Brooks-Gordon, B., Esin, C., Holt, A., Mehdizadeh, L. and Shinebourne, P. (2010) Pluralism in qualitative research. *Qualitative Research* 10(4), 441–460. https://doi.org/10.1177/1468794110366802

Garcia Pinillos, R., Appleby, M.C., Manteca, X., Scott-Park, F., Smith, C. and Velarde, A. (2016) One welfare – a platform for improving human and animal welfare. *Veterinary Record* 179, 412–413. doi:10.1136/vr.i5470

Ghai, R. (2014) Kartick Satyanarayan, the man who made an elephant weep with joy. *Business Standard*. Available at: https://www.business-standard.com/article/beyond-business/kartick-satyanarayan-the-man-who-made-an-elephant-weep-with-joy-114072500654_1.html (accessed 9 April 2021).

Hawkins, R.D., Williams, J.M. and Scottish Society for the Prevention of Cruelty to Animals (2017) Assessing effectiveness of a nonhuman animal welfare education program for primary school children. *Journal of Applied Animal Welfare Science* 20(3), 240–256. doi:10.1080/10888705.2017.1305272

International Animal Rescue (2009) Animal welfare history is made as the final curtain falls on dancing bears in India. Available at: https://www.internationalanimalrescue.org/news/animal-welfare-history-made-final-curtain-falls-dancing-bears-india (accessed 9 April 2021).

Lebedko, M. (2013) Theory and practice of stereotypes in intercultural communication. In Houghton, S.A., Furumura, Y., Lebedko, M. and Li, S. (eds) *Critical Cultural Awareness*. Cambridge Scholars Publishing, Cambridge, UK, 4–23.

Mburu, S., Zaibet, L., Fall, A. and Ndiwa, N. (2012) The role of working animals in the livelihoods of rural communities in West Africa. Livestock Research for Rural Development 24, article 156. Available at: www.lrrd.org/lrrd24/9/mbur24156.htm (accessed 9 April 2021).

Mengjie, W. and Yi, D. (1996) The importance of work animals in rural China. *World Animal Review* 86, 1996/1, FAO, Rome. Available at: www.fao.org/3/w0613t/w0613T0p.htm#the importance of work animals in rural china (accessed 9 April 2021).

Mitra, D. and Valette, D. (2017) Brick by brick: Environment, human labour and animal welfare. International Labour Organization, The Brooke Hospital for Animals and The Donkey Sanctuary. Available at: https://www.thebrooke.org/sites/default/files/Downloads/Brick%20by%20Brick%20report.pdf (accessed 9 April 2021).

Moorhouse, T.P., Dahlsjö, C.A.L., Baker, S.E., D'Cruze, N.C. and Macdonald, D.W. (2015) The customer isn't always right – conservation and animal welfare implications of the increasing demand for wildlife tourism. *PLoS ONE* 10(10), e0138939. https://doi.org/10.1371/journal.pone.0138939

Pollock, P.J. (2018) Working equids in refugee camps. Forced Migration Review, June 2018, 7–8. Available at: https://www.fmreview.org/sites/fmr/files/FMRdownloads/en/economies/humans-animals-camps.pdf (accessed 9 April 2021).

Pritchard, J.C., Lindberg, A.C., Main, D.C.J. and Whay, H.R. (2005) Assessment of the welfare of working horses, mules and donkeys, using health and behaviour parameters. *Preventative Veterinary Medicine* 69(3–4), 265–283. https://doi.org/10.1016/j.prevetmed.2005.02.002

Reuveny, R. (2007) Climate change-induced migration and violent conflict. *Political Geography* 26, 656–673.

Schaul, J.C. (2012) Wildlife SOS-India nearly extinguishes a 400-year-old practice of dancing bears. *National Geographic*. Available at: https://blog.nationalgeographic.org/2012/10/11/wildlife-sos-india-nearly-extinguishes-a-400-year-old-practice-of-dancing-bears (accessed 9 April 2021).

Sommerville, R., Brown, A.F. and Upjohn, M. (2018) A standardised equine-based welfare assessment tool used for six years in low and middle income countries. *PLoS ONE*, e0192354. https://doi.org/10.1371/journal.pone.0192354

SPANA (2020) Homepage. Available at: https://spana.org (accessed 9 April 2021).

Swai, E.S. and Bwanga, S.J.R. (2008) Donkey keeping in northern Tanzania: Socio-economic roles and reported husbandry and health constraints. *Livestock Research for Rural Development* 20(5), article 67. Available at: www.lrrd.org/lrrd20/5/swai20067.htm (accessed 9 April 2021).

Swann, W. (2006) Improving the welfare of working equine animals in developing countries. *Applied Animal Behaviour* Science 100(1–2), 148–151. https://doi.org/10.1016/j.applanim.2006.04.001

Tourism Concern (2017) Animals in tourism, research briefing. Available at: https://www.tourismconcern.org.uk/wp-content/uploads/2018/03/Animals-in-Tourism-lWeb-FINAL-1.pdf (accessed 9 April 2021).

Valette, D. (2014) Invisible helpers. Voices from women international report. Brooke. Available at: https://www.thebrooke.org/sites/default/files/Advocacy-and-policy/Invisible-helpers-voices-from-women.pdf (accessed 9 April 2021).

van Dijk, L., Pritchard, J., Pradhan, S.K. and Wells, K. (2011) Sharing the load: A guide to improving the welfare of working animals through collective action. Practical Action Publishing, Rugby, UK.

Wemelsfelder, F. and Mullan, S. (2014) Applying ethological and health indicators to practical animal welfare assessment. *OIE Scientific and Technical Review* 33(1), 111–120.

Werrell, C.E. and Femia, F. (2018) Climate change raises conflict concerns. The UNESCO Courier, 2018-2. Available at: https://en.unesco.org/courier/2018-2/climate-change-raises-conflict-concerns (accessed 9 April 2021).

Wildlife SOS (2019) A conservation success: celebrating 10 years of India's last 'Dancing Bear' rescue! Available at: https://wildlifesos.org/animals/a-conservation-success-celebrating-10-years-of-indias-last-dancing-bear-rescue (accessed 9 April 2021).

World Animal Net (2017) Working animals. Animal Welfare Issues. Available at: https://worldanimal.net/documents/6_Working_Animals.pdf (accessed 9 April 2021).

11 Strengthening Existing Healthcare Systems for Sustainable Animal Welfare

Shereene Williams and Laura Skippen
Brooke Action for Working Horses and Donkeys, London, UK

11.1 Introduction

The health of an animal is inextricably linked with its welfare. An animal that is diseased, injured or in pain cannot be considered to be in a positive welfare state at that point. It is impossible to prevent every instance of disease or injury; therefore, access to good-quality preventative care and treatment is a vital component of animal welfare. The World Health Organization (WHO, 1946) states that 'The enjoyment of the highest attainable standard of health is one of the fundamental rights of every human being without distinction of race, religion, political belief, economic or social condition' and this right is just as vital for animals. As with people, the reality is very different for many animals depending on their role and where they live. A well-functioning health system is built on having trained and motivated health workers, a well-maintained infrastructure, and a reliable supply of medicines and technologies, backed by adequate funding, strong health plans and evidence-based policies (WHO, 2020b), and this definition works equally for animal health systems (Fig. 11.1). Beyond the behaviour change of individuals, systemic changes are needed to improve animal welfare.

11.2 Work and Life as an Animal Welfare Practitioner

Laura and Shereene are veterinary surgeons who lead the Global Animal Health (GAH) UK team at Brooke Action for Working Horses and Donkeys (Brooke), working alongside international colleagues across Brooke programmes in Africa, Asia, the Middle East and Latin America. Brooke strengthens local animal health services by training and mentoring local vets, veterinary paraprofessionals and farriers. The GAH teams within each country are made up of

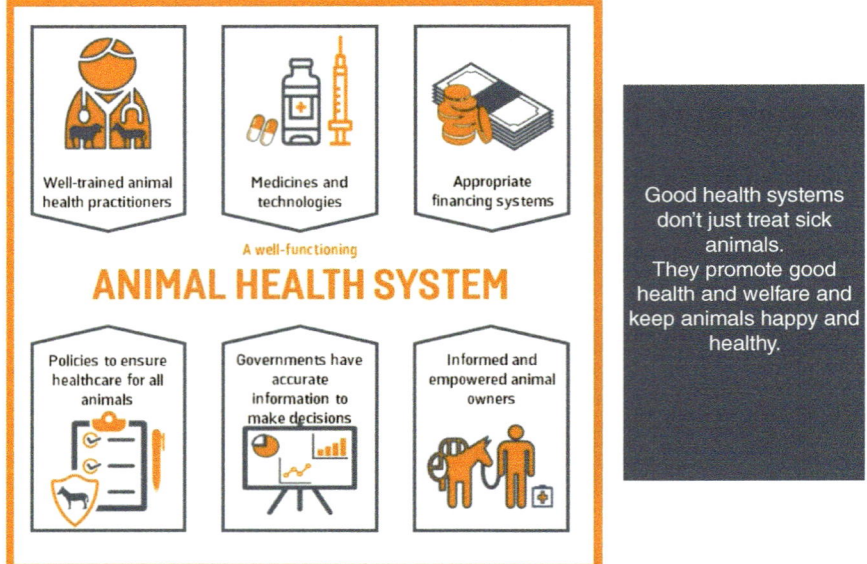

Fig. 11.1. A well-functioning animal health system. (© Brooke, 2021.)

local veterinarians who have the most direct practical experience to carry out healthcare mentoring and lead local initiatives, as well as inputting their local knowledge into global projects. The UK team lead cross-cutting projects that have been developed around prioritized welfare issues in the health systems globally; for example, access to essential medicine, training and legislation of veterinary paraprofessionals – practitioners with variable qualifications and length of training who deliver the majority of veterinary services in rural low- and middle-income countries (LMIC), legally under the supervision of a qualified vet (Ouma, 2015) and professionalization of farriery. Both authors spend extensive time in the field supporting teams in developing mentoring skills and planning interventions on key welfare issues (Fig. 11.2).

Laura qualified from the Royal Veterinary College, London in 2005. Throughout her university time she travelled extensively, spent time working for VetAid in Mozambique, completed overseas placements as part of final year rotations and represented the university in animal welfare forums. On graduating Laura went into general equine practice in the UK and worked closely with the Royal Society for the Prevention of Cruelty to Animals (RSPCA) and the Donkey Sanctuary, gaining experience of collaborating with owners and other animal welfare professionals to improve the lives of animals in UK cruelty cases. Laura joined Brooke in 2012 running practical training on equine health and welfare for Brooke's vets.

Having completing a PGCert in veterinary education, Laura focuses on improving education in veterinary training institutions, alongside capacity building Brooke's current workforce through the Animal Health Mentoring Framework. Encouraging adoption of international guidelines such as the World

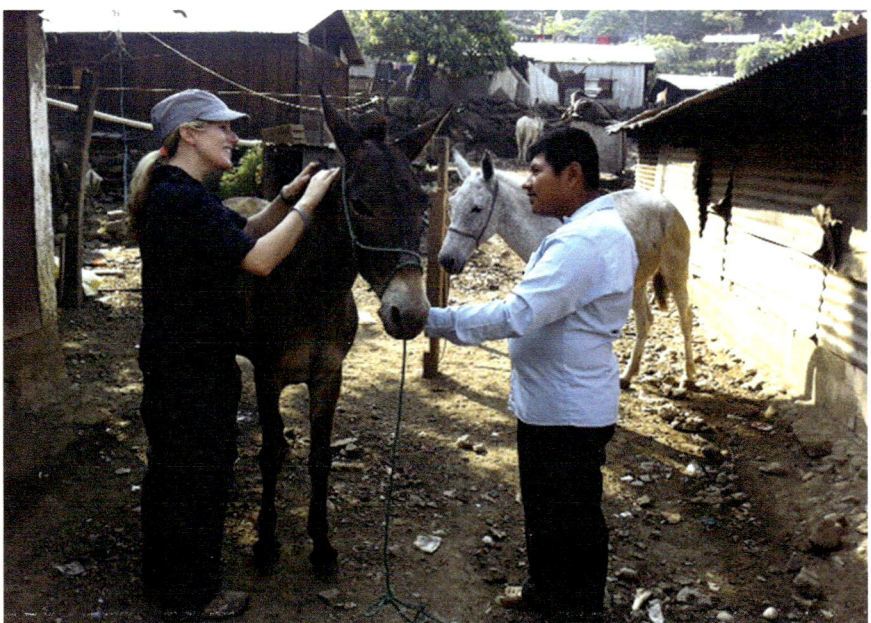

Fig. 11.2. Author Laura carrying out welfare appraisal with a mule and his owner in Chiapas, Mexico.

Organisation for Animal Health (OIE) Day One Competencies for Veterinary Paraprofessionals (OIE, 2018) and associated curriculum guidelines (OIE, 2019) are an effective way to ensure that animal welfare, practical handling skills and improved clinical skills are central in the future education for veterinary paraprofessionals globally; a crucial step towards more animals having access to competent, compassionate veterinary paraprofessionals acting as advocates for their health, as a domain of welfare.

Shereene, from a young age, spent time with her father's family in Sri Lanka and there first understood the plight of animals within LMICs forming her desire to work with and help animals. Shereene qualified in 2011 from Nottingham Veterinary School, UK. She started her career at welfare organization Redwings Horse Sanctuary in the centre's hospital. She also worked alongside the RSPCA and other charities to provide veterinary and welfare support to marginalized owners and their equids.

After a few busy years in rural mixed veterinary practice in the UK, Shereene traded her stethoscope for a backpack and travelled across Asia and Africa, further enhancing her desire to work to sustainably improve animal welfare in LMICs. Shereene returned to practice in Australia before joining Brooke in 2016. Shereene completed further qualifications in medical education and is currently working towards a Master's in One Health at the University of Edinburgh. Shereene focuses on building mentoring skills in vets and farriers, and leads Brooke's Global Farriery Project aiming

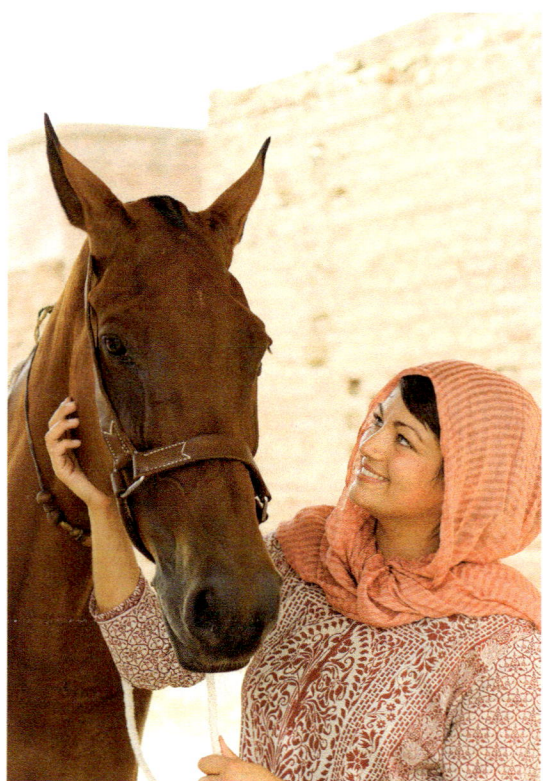

Fig. 11.3. Author Shereene alongside a hard-working horse in Faisalabad, Pakistan.

to address the critical welfare issues of lameness and hoof pain. Shereene also works to improve access to essential medicines and believes it is only when vets and veterinary paraprofessionals work within a system that supports them to access the necessary resources that they can use their skills and knowledge to provide quality care for animals and make lasting change (Fig. 11.3).

11.3 Improving Animal Welfare as an Equine Welfare NGO

11.3.1 How does good animal health enable good animal welfare?

It is clear how the health of an animal can impact its own welfare, but how does the health of a population of animals and access to a good-quality animal health system improve an animal's lifetime experience?

Consider the fatal zoonotic disease rabies. Rabies is an entirely preventable disease in humans and animals; however, the coveted rabies-free status is almost entirely reserved for higher income countries (HICs) with strong animal health systems. The risks of fatal zoonotic diseases have taught humans to fear animals, to protect themselves and their property from them, and even to object to their very existence. Looking at the statistic for rabies, these can be interpreted as justified fears. Rabies is estimated to cause 59,000 deaths annually in more than 150 countries, and 95% of deaths occur in Africa and Asia (WHO, 2020a). The burden of disease is disproportionally felt by rural poor communities. Around 99% of cases are dog mediated (OIE, 2020).

This learnt fear of animals has passed through generations for millennia and results in many practices that are detrimental to animal welfare; that is, physical abuse, forced expulsion and even mass culling programmes. While people fear for their own health existing alongside animals, it is hard to believe that a truly positive relationship between the two can be realized.

Ensuring that animals pose no or minimal disease threat to humans and that this is well communicated through trusted animal health professionals is essential to promote a positive relationship between animals and people and therefore vital in ensuring good animal welfare.

11.3.2 Animal healthcare providers are animal welfare advocates

Animal healthcare providers have a critical role to play as animal welfare advocates. In an HIC context an animal owner has many people to seek help from: vets, nurses, behaviourists, farriers and other paraprofessionals, who can all be a source of expert animal health advice. In an LMIC context, a veterinary paraprofessional, community animal health worker or traditional healer may be the only source of advice for miles around. While animal owners play the most critical day-to-day role in the life of an animal, when they do need help the person providing that help must act as the voice of the animal and model compassionate treatment, as discussed in Chapter 10. In many contexts animal healthcare providers are well-respected community members. Demonstrating empathy and belief in the importance of good animal welfare is a vital method in bringing animal owners on the same journey.

11.3.3 Policy changes to recognize working animals

Working livestock, animals providing draft power and transport primarily rather than food-producing, are frequently overlooked in policy in favour of food-producing livestock. They often do not have the same protection under animal welfare laws or the same investment into their healthcare. Yet an estimated 500 million people in LMICs rely on donkeys as a source of income (Brooke, 2015; Fig. 11.4).

Developing evidence for the importance of working animals and their connection to bettering human livelihoods is key to ensuring their place

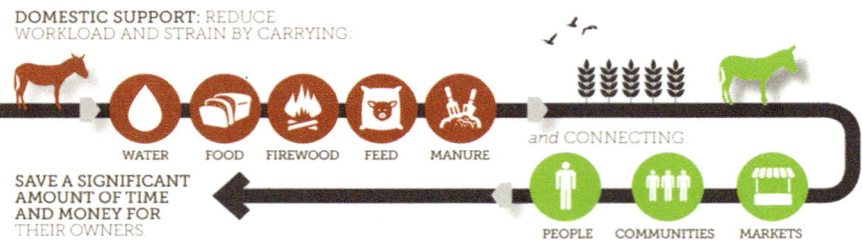

Fig. 11.4. How working equids contribute to people's livelihoods all around the world. (© Brooke, 2015.)

in government policy and therefore securing funding for better health and welfare. Healthy and happy animals support healthy and happy people. This is particularly true for women and children, who are most reliant on working animals for relieving the household workload, thereby keeping children in school and allowing women to earn income elsewhere. Understanding where existing policy can be reworked to include an invisible sector, thus gaining recognition and rights, is essential when looking at the whole system. Long-term advocacy for working equids to be termed as 'working livestock' has improved their visibility and their access to government health schemes.

11.3.4 Healthcare in remote settings

Last-mile healthcare in human medicine has no formal definition but is a term for the delivery of primary healthcare services (e.g. vaccinations, maternal care, neonatal) delivered to remote, rural communities many miles from formal healthcare settings (Last Mile Health, 2020). Last-mile animal healthcare is very similar. Animals and their owners in remote communities often do not have the transport or funds to access qualified healthcare professionals. It falls to those with little training or support to provide routine preventative and emergency care for the animals that provide a lifeline in these settings. Local animal healthcare providers are usually veterinary paraprofessionals or community animal health workers with training varying from a couple of years to a few weeks. With minimal training, mostly theory-based in line with current practices in training institutions, they face the same complex health issues that challenge well-qualified vets. Animal healthcare providers are also constrained by a lack of access to medicines, scarce diagnostic tests and weak referral systems for specialist support from other professionals. Finally, they may be legally limited in what services they can provide, as their registration requirements and legal status varies hugely across the globe. Despite these limitations, it is essential to recognize that some form of healthcare will exist in nearly all communities; identifying who is providing it (e.g. local pharmacist, traditional healer) and who is using it is the first step towards being able to strengthen a health system.

11.3.5 Sustainable healthcare support from NGOs

Historically animal welfare focused non-governmental organizations (NGOs) working in LMICs have approached the problem of poor-quality healthcare by setting up new systems (e.g. drop-in clinics for animal owners) offering high-quality, free or low-cost healthcare which then undermines the system that was in place, however poor that system may have been. This is not sustainable long term; if a foreign entity is providing free or subsidized healthcare then there is always the risk that this will be withdrawn if there are legal or security issues, there is a reduction in funding or the NGO's priorities change. Instead building the capacity of those within the local healthcare system and building demand for their services from animal owners simultaneously is a more viable approach for NGOs to support. Creating a functional privatized system means that both the skills and the use of those skills by animal owners will remain in the area even when external support is withdrawn. If the aim is to create a good-quality healthcare system, then all the aspects mentioned in Fig. 11.1 must be addressed locally to ensure that the system will remain working for future generations of animals.

Developing an existing animal health system into a unit of confident, competent, compassionate animal health practitioners who are accessible and affordable for animal owners, and who have access to good-quality medicines and resources, including diagnostics, is only half the battle. If animal owners are not also brought on the same journey so that they value their animals highly enough to seek improved services and are willing to pay for preventative and curative treatments, then the best health system will fail. Human behaviour change is a critical component of strengthening animal health systems, both in creating animal welfare advocates in the workforce who will speak up for the benefit of the animal, and to encourage owners to appreciate and use the improved system and imitate the behaviour they see from their animal healthcare provider.

11.4 Overcoming Challenges

Based on field experience the authors identify challenges common to animal health systems in LMICs. The following case studies highlight three key issues routinely encountered by those trying to strengthen existing animal health systems: lack of available good-quality healthcare providers, ensuring prioritization of animal health services and access to essential, good-quality medicines. These case studies demonstrate sustainable ways of working to build local workforce capacity and create profitable businesses and supply chains, while also addressing crucial welfare needs for working animals.

Case Study 1: Reaching More Animals by Treating Fewer in Pakistan

Pakistan has one of the largest populations of working equids in Asia at 5.9 million (Brooke, 2018; Fig. 11.5). Working equids support people to earn a living by transporting people and goods, collecting water, working within agriculture and construction. Common health and welfare conditions include lameness, abnormal hoof shape, poor body condition, wounds and eye disease (Brooke, 2018).

Historically, Brooke Pakistan employed a direct service provision model, involving 25 vets, 3 hospitals and 28 mobile veterinary treatment vehicles. The team treated on average 156,000 animals a year, providing free medicines and valuable advice, resulting in high-quality veterinary care and close relationships with animal owners.

Challenges arose when considering the sustainability and reach of this model. While effective in providing high-quality care for a small number, without increasing resources proportionally there was no hope of reaching all of the working equids. The goal of improving animal welfare had inadvertently created a parallel system with reliance on Brooke for maintenance. For all working equids within Pakistan to have access to quality, affordable healthcare the delivery mechanism had to change.

In 2016, Brooke Pakistan stopped free treatments and focused efforts on strengthening the existing animal healthcare system. In particular they focused on ensuring access to confident, compassionate, competent animal health providers. Vets ceased providing treatments except in emergencies, identified existing animal healthcare providers within a community, often paravets, and started mentoring and training them. Globally paravet training and regulation is weak. Training varies from 2 weeks to 2 years leading to varying levels of competency among them and harmful practices, such as misdiagnosis, blanket treatments, poor clinical skills and harmful handling.

Brooke highlighted five essential competency areas:

- animal welfare;
- communication;
- clinical expertize;
- kit contents and maintenance; and
- clinical governance.

Brooke created the Animal Health Mentoring Framework (Brooke, 2020), a checklist of competencies and essential equipment and medicines needed in order to provide quality healthcare. This trains mentors in how to support and coach providers through cases on the job; a practical approach for individuals who often have low literacy and competency levels.

Continued

Case Study 1: Continued.

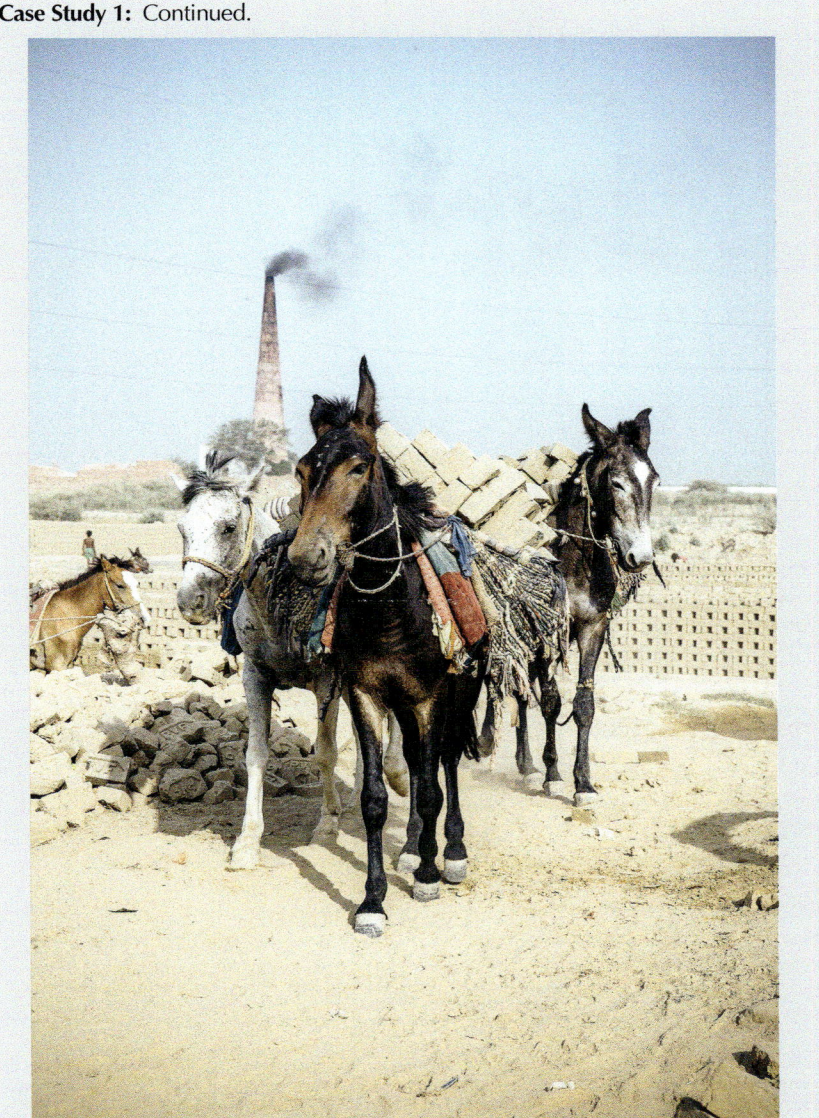

Fig. 11.5. Working equids in the brick kilns of Pakistan. (© Brooke, 2016.)

Baseline data determined the existing competency of the selected providers and informed a training needs assessment for a programme of monthly mentoring, prioritizing important health issues. Quantitative and qualitative data were collected and analysed quarterly to inform ongoing mentoring.

A significant improvement (35%) in overall competencies (Fig. 11.3) was observed after 1 year. Practitioners were more confident and competent to approach, handle and restrain equids in a welfare-friendly way. Their clinical reasoning and

Continued

Case Study 1: Continued.

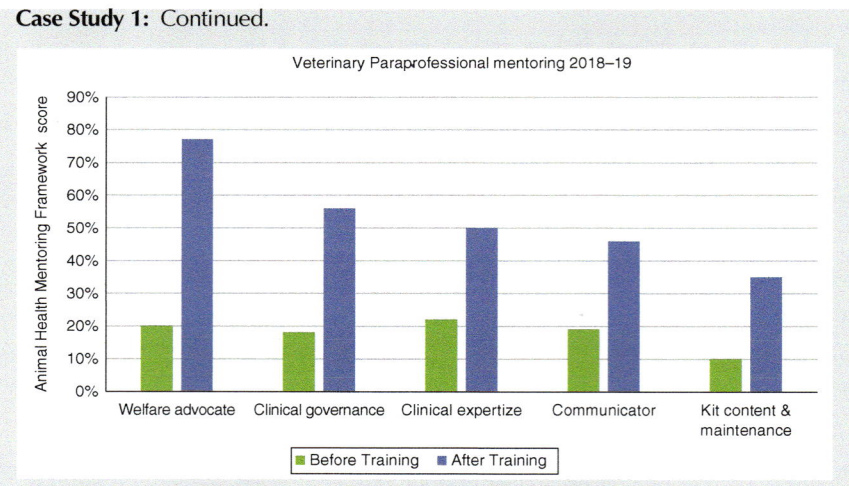

Fig. 11.6. Veterinary paraprofessional mentoring in Pakistan 2018–2019.

practical skills improved and they were more assertive in disseminating preventative health and husbandry messages to owners. These skills will remain within communities without intensive support from Brooke (Fig. 11.6).

Dr Javed Gondal, Programme Manager of Brooke Pakistan (personal communication) notes:

Instead of treating animals ourselves, our approach to strengthen the existing animal health system and focus on training local Animal Healthcare Providers improves health and welfare for more animals. Working with local providers and marginalized equine owning communities, we are building lasting skills, developing compassion and care towards all animals. Previously we reached 150,000 animals a year providing free treatments. Now we work with owners to develop self-reliance and problem-solving skills and link them with trained local Animal Healthcare Providers. Additionally we advocate for national changes in animal welfare policies. We now reach over 560,000 animals. We encourage others to prioritise existing local knowledge and practices and build sustainable support structures in the form of local groups for collective action.

Case Study 2: One Welfare Livestock Programmes in Afghanistan

Afghanistan is one of the poorest countries in the world; 54% of the population live below the poverty line. A total of 74.8% of the population live in rural areas, mostly dependent on agriculture and livestock for their livelihoods. Afghanistan has suffered many wars with disastrous consequences for the animal healthcare system, including destruction of the national veterinary school, and the collapse of government veterinary services. The challenge of rebuilding an animal healthcare system from scratch with few resources and poor infrastructure was enormous.

Continued

Case Study 2: Continued.

Dutch Committee for Afghanistan (DCA) asked communities to highlight their most pressing livestock issues. Farmers identified livestock losses to disease, a lack of knowledge on animal husbandry and nutrition, and few market opportunities for livestock products. To address the problems related to animal health and ensure that farmers had access to trained service providers who provided husbandry and nutrition advice, a network of competent veterinary paraprofessionals, who would be well accepted by their own communities, needed to be trained. Graduate professionals at the time were few in number and poorly educated.

DCA developed a successful model using trained veterinary paraprofessionals working in Veterinary Field Units (field clinics) and a network of 800 Veterinary Field Units was established across Afghanistan. Paraprofessional trainees are recruited from their local community in consultation with the Shura (community leaders). This selection process ensures that veterinary paraprofessionals are accepted by the community and want to work in the area. A trainee receives 24 weeks' practical training from DCA training centres on animal handling, husbandry, disease diagnosis and treatment. They are then set up in a Veterinary Field Unit in their local community, usually close to a livestock market or village centre, to deliver high-quality mobile and static services to all livestock species. These are fee-paying services so the business can become self-sufficient after 1–2 years. During this time DCA staff members continue to mentor the new paravet and ensure they receive ongoing training to increase their skills and the services they can offer.

Each Veterinary Field Unit must establish an extension group of at least ten livestock owners in two villages. Extension activities by the paravets promote their own businesses but also give health and welfare advice to farmers, both male and female, thus fulfilling the second challenge identified by communities.

When Brooke identified Afghanistan as a country with a working equid population in extreme need, rather than setting up a parallel project to focus solely on equids, it went into partnership with DCA, already a well-respected NGO with a functioning system in place. DCA has included equine welfare training, including humane handling, in their veterinary paraprofessional curriculum, meaning that all those recently trained are able to treat working equids compassionately and advocate for their welfare. Most veterinary paraprofessionals spend the majority of their working lives treating other livestock species; an approach focusing only on one species would not have been economically worthwhile for them to be involved in.

In a country where the human population has suffered so much, an approach focused solely on the welfare of animals would be untenable and insensitive. However, by including welfare of animals as part of a programme to improve animal health and productivity for the benefit of human livelihoods it has become normalized in the system. Recently the Afghan Ministry of Labour certified the DCA training of veterinary paraprofessionals; welfare and compassionate handling is now included in training for all veterinary paraprofessionals in Afghanistan. Welfare is not the sole focus of the project, but its inclusion within a project that has benefits for humans too means it is being more widely promoted. By linking animal welfare to human health and wellbeing priorities, DCA has succeeded in mainstreaming animal welfare, pioneering a One Welfare approach.

Case Study 3: Knowledge Alone Cannot Relieve Pain in East Africa

Brooke East Africa (BEA) is based in Kenya, and works through partners in Tanzania, Somaliland and South Sudan (Fig. 11.7).

A priority welfare issue is the recognition and relief of pain. Planned training covered basic concepts; however, applying this in the field was a significant challenge for animal healthcare providers. Through mentoring and group training

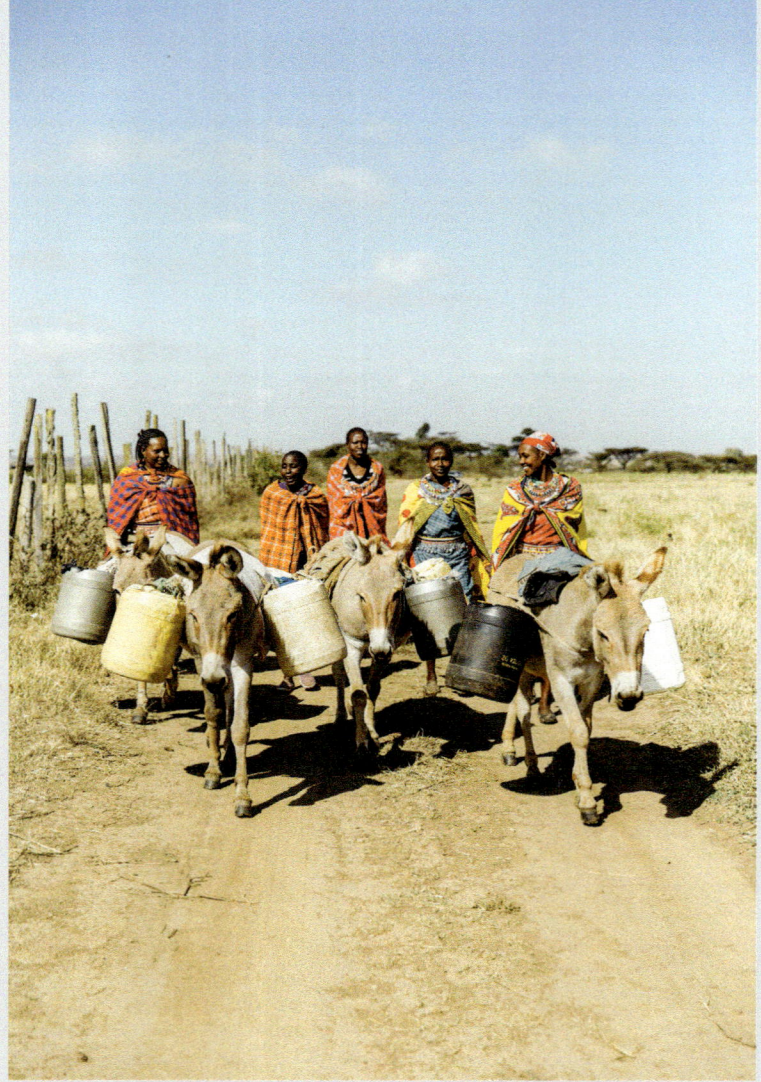

Fig. 11.7. Maasai women collecting water with their donkeys, Kenya. (© Brooke, 2016.)

Continued

Case Study 3: Continued.

conducted by BEA, skills and knowledge were built in vets and paravets. However, on review, BEA felt that this had not translated into pain being recognized and managed to an acceptable level for animals in the field.

BEA asked over 3000 owners one question: 'What do you do when your animal gets sick?' A total of 70% of respondents said that they visited a local agrovet to seek advice and get medication. It became clear that agrovets (agriculture and veterinary drug stores run by paraprofessionals) play a key role in primary animal healthcare. A study (Onono and Kithuka, 2020) into agrovet ways of working confirmed approximately 50% were qualified and licensed; therefore, many were poorly equipped with the technical knowledge to dispense medicine and offer advice.

BEA incorporated agrovets into an adapted version of the established training and mentoring system, which was successful in developing competence in recognition of pain. However, the administration of pain relief medicines remained rare. In working closely with the agrovets the team realized that pain relief medicines, such as non-steroidal anti-inflammatory drugs (NSAIDs), were not stocked in the shops. This corresponded to minimal availability of NSAIDs within veterinary practitioners' kits, highlighting a systemic unavailability. While the skills to recognize and treat pain were now present, animals were still not receiving the relief they needed, translating to unnecessary animal suffering and a negative welfare state.

To address this, a partnership with the organization Sidai was formed. Sidai is a social enterprise in Kenya, set up by Farm Africa to supply quality livestock medicines and resources to farmers and pastoralists via a network of franchised retail outlets.

The project held discussions with 445 animal health practitioners to understand their views and the field realities. Tailored technical training for service providers focusing on the value of pain management and work within the supply chain ensured that all Sidai hubs stocked one form of pain relief that could be used for equids and all livestock. Large-scale promotion of animal welfare, including pain relief and its benefits for all species, took place with farmers, service providers and agrovets. The team also monitored stock levels and the uptake of pain relief within target areas (Fig. 11.8).

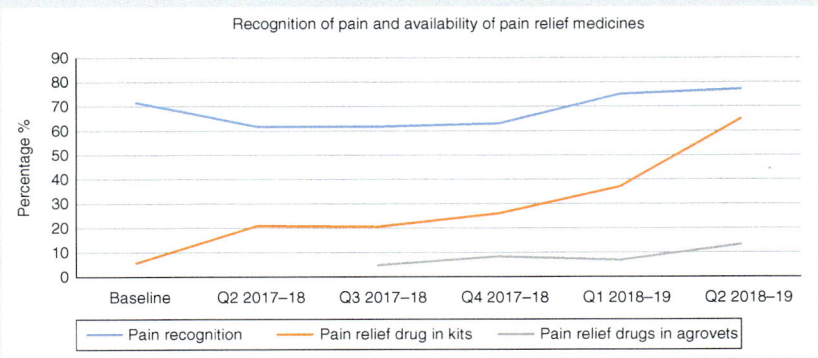

Fig. 11.8. Recognition of pain and availability of pain relief medicines in East Africa 2017–2019.

Continued

Case Study 3: Continued.

These synchronized activities resulted in a corresponding increase in presence of pain relief in practitioners' kits – an increase in 60% from the baseline. Interestingly pain recognition by providers also improved compared with when there was no availability.

To address complex welfare issues such as pain caused by a lack of access to essential medicines, it is not enough to concentrate solely on knowledge and skill of one set of stakeholders. Systemic issues require a multi-stakeholder approach addressing all aspects of the supply chain from registration to distribution and uptake. Working in partnership with those who can lobby and advocate for sustainable change that can be implemented locally is essential. Quick fixes, such as one international NGO importing and distributing essential medicines, will not result in a sustained change for animal welfare. All stakeholders from the farmers, vets and paravets, medicine merchants, veterinary and government bodies should be engaged ensuring that both demand and a sustainable supply are in place.

How to Change the Behaviour of Animal Healthcare Providers in LMICs

- Animal health is not just the absence of disease; it is about sustaining animals in a positive welfare state. Prevention, via positive welfare, is better than cure.
- Veterinary paraprofessionals are key animal welfare advocates. Within LMICs they may be the only source of trusted welfare advice that can be accessed by owners.
- Always ask the question 'What do you do when your animal gets sick?' to investigate the existing system when commencing any intervention.
- Try and look beyond the animal in front of you and consider the whole system in which that animal exists.
- Aim to improve the lives of a population of animals, not just an individual.
- Learn from experience outside the animal healthcare world, e.g. human medicine, social care, education. Many challenges will be similar and lessons can be learnt.
- Animal health and welfare matters to more than just animals; link animal welfare to other global priorities by looking for opportunities to partner with ongoing successful initiatives, e.g. through the framework of the Sustainable Development Goals.
- Work with owners to create demand for good quality services alongside developing animal healthcare systems to ensure these remain sustainable in the long term.

11.5 Conclusions

Animal health and animal welfare have often been separated, with healthcare focused on prevention and treatment of specific diseases, and good welfare considered as an absence of negative occurrences. As welfare has developed to consider aspects of positive welfare and 'a life worth living' (Mellor, 2017,

p. 60), so healthcare has developed to consider broader definitions of disease, including mental wellbeing and quality of life, which are included in One Health (WHO, 2017). To attain the highest level of animal welfare possible we need to ensure strong animal health systems globally. This cannot be done by veterinarians alone. Governments, policy makers, training/research institutions, health and welfare professionals must collaborate and support those who have the most impact on animals' lifetime experiences, and whose animals' health and welfare is inextricably linked to their own, namely veterinary paraprofessionals and owners.

An animal in a positive welfare state is more resilient to disease and more likely to have a life worth living. Existing in a positive welfare state helps ensure animals are effective in their role and can support their owners' lives and livelihoods. Therefore, animal welfare is essential to the 1.3 billion people globally who depend on livestock for their livelihoods (ILRI, 2020). Working alongside owners to build skills and knowledge, while learning about system limitations, ensures that local and national advocacy campaigns and policies are well informed and positioned to make real change for those on the ground. Evidencing links is vital for animal welfare to become a priority issue and benefit from increased visibility and funding.

Whether global policy or field-level interventions, it is critical to look beyond the visible issue and consider the whole system in which animals and people exist. Well-intentioned kneejerk reactions, such as providing free veterinary treatment or importing medicines, may provide short-term relief or improvement to a few animals, but an artificial system that does not address the root cause cannot be sustained, and will never make the large-scale impact that we know is needed.

Summary

More can be achieved by working with what is already in place, compared with creating new systems that undermine local systems and traditions. However, creating lasting improvements in animal health systems at a national level is an ambitious task. Last-mile human healthcare is a key issue in the drive to achieve universal health coverage (WHO, 2020b) for all people and looking to the ways that humanitarian agencies are trying to achieve this will be key in driving this forwards for all animals in the future. To push animal welfare up the global agenda and create a catalyst for change, referencing solely animal welfare is not enough. Drawing on linkages between people, the planet and animals is essential.

11.6 Recommended Resources

- Brooke's Animal Health Mentoring Framework, https://www.thebrooke.org/our-work/brookes-animal-health-mentoring-framework (accessed 12 April 2020).

- Using a One Health approach, https://www.thebrooke.org/our-work/one-health-brooke (accessed 12 April 2020).
- World Organisation for Animal Health, https://www.oie.int (accessed 12 April 2020).
- World Organisation for Animal Health working equid standards videos, https://www.youtube.com/playlist?list=PLWxqgr70i8RtSNbjix7fnTnXoG-19LQhl (accessed 12 April 2020).
- International Coalition for Working Equids, https://www.icweworkingequids.org (accessed 12 April 2020).
- Dutch Committee for Afghanistan, https://dca-livestock.org (accessed 12 April 2020).
- World Health Organization constitution, https://www.who.int/about/who-we-are/constitution (accessed 12 April 2020).
- World Health Organization universal health coverage, https://www.who.int/news-room/fact-sheets/detail/universal-health-coverage-(uhc) (accessed 12 April 2020).
- International Livestock Research Institute, https://www.ilri.org (accessed 12 April 2020).
- Action for Animal Health, https://actionforanimalhealth.org (accessed 12 April 2020).
- Sidai Africa Limited, https://www.sidai.com (accessed 12 April 2020).
- United Nations Sustainable Development Goals, https://www.undp.org/content/undp/en/home/sustainable-development-goals.html#:~:text=The%20Sustainable%20Development%20Goals%20(SDGs,peace%20and%20prosperity%20by%202030 (accessed 12 April 2020).

Acknowledgements

With special thanks to Dr Javed Gondal, Dr James Kithuka and Dr Raymond Briscoe for their contributions to the featured case studies. Thank you to Brooke colleagues, past and present, whose collective passion drives learning and improves animal welfare in some of the most challenging circumstances. The views and opinions expressed in this chapter are those of the authors and do not necessarily reflect the position of any other organization.

References

Brooke Action for Working Horses and Donkeys (2015) Invisible workers. Available at: https://www.thebrooke.org/sites/default/files/Advocacy-and-policy/Invisible-workers-report-2020.pdf (accessed 1 September 2020).
Brooke Action for Working Horses and Donkeys (2018) Pakistan at a glance. Available at: https://www.thebrooke.org/our-work/pakistan (accessed 22 November 2020).

Brooke Action for Working Horses and Donkeys (2020) Brookes Animal Health Mentoring Framework. Available at: https://www.thebrooke.org/our-work/brookes-animal-health-mentoring-framework (accessed 22 November 2020).

International Livestock Research Institute (ILRI) (2020) Prosperity. Available at: https://www.ilri.org/research/themes/prosperity (accessed 30 November 2020).

Last Mile Health (2020) What we do. Available at: https://lastmilehealth.org/what-we-do (accessed 30 November 2020).

Mellor, D.J. (2017) Operational details of the Five Domains Models and its key applications to the assessment and management of animal welfare. *Animals* 7(8), 60. doi:10.3390/ani7080060

Onono, O. and Kithuka, J. (2020) Assessment of provision of extension services and advocacy on donkey health and welfare in Kenya. *Asian Journal of Agricultural Extension, Economics and Sociology* 38(5), 15–28. doi:10.9734/AJAEES/2020/v38i530344

Ouma, B. (2015) Recognising the vital role of veterinary paraprofessionals. Available at: https://www.galvmed.org/recognising-the-vital-role-of-veterinary-paraprofessionals (accessed 1 December 2020).

World Health Organization (WHO) (1946) Constitution. Available at: https://www.who.int/about/who-we-are/constitution (accessed 6 December 2020).

World Health Organization (WHO) (2017) What is 'One Health'? Available at: https://www.who.int/news-room/q-a-detail/one-health#:~:text='One%20Health'%20is%20an%20approach,achieve%20better%20public%20health%20outcomes (accessed 17 October 2020).

World Health Organization (WHO) (2020a) Rabies: key facts. Available at: https://www.who.int/news-room/fact-sheets/detail/rabies (accessed 26 October 2020).

World Health Organization (WHO) (2020b) Universal health coverage. Available at: https://www.who.int/health-topics/universal-health-coverage#tab=tab_1 (accessed 7 December 2020).

World Organisation for Animal Health (OIE) (2018) OIE competency guidelines for veterinary paraprofessionals. Available at: https://www.oie.int/fileadmin/Home/eng/Support_to_OIE_Members/docs/pdf/A_Competence.pdf (accessed 30 November 2020).

World Organisation for Animal Health (OIE) (2019) OIE curricula guidelines for veterinary paraprofessionals. Available at: https://www.oie.int/fileadmin/Home/eng/Support_to_OIE_Members/docs/pdf/AF-CoreCV-ANG.pdf (accessed 30 November 2020).

World Organisation for Animal Health (OIE) (2020) Rabies still kills. Available at: https://www.oie.int/en/animal-health-in-the-world/rabies-portal (accessed 3 October 2020).

Index

Note: The page numbers in bold and italics represents tables and figures respectively.

active learning 72
African swine fever (ASF) 100
amygdala 41
anchoring biases 38
animal welfare
    approaches 6, **14–17**
    broiler chickens 8
    captive whales/dolphins 6–7
    choked cat 10
    communications 40–41
    curriculum *see* curriculum
    definition 2
    domains 3, **4**
    education 65–69
    engagement/campaigning 8
    formal training 5
    India *see* India
    initiate a community 62
    nature of working 36
    NGO
        animal health interventions 87
        battery cages 84–85, *85*
        commercial broiler
            chickens 86, 87
        egg industry 84
        factory farming model 86
        farm animals endure 84
        gestation 85, 86
        higher-welfare systems 87
        narrowing efforts 84
        organizations 85
        prevalence 84
        smallholders 86
        smallholdings 87
    practitioner 1, 5, **5**
    rabbits 11–12, *12*
    three spheres framework *36*
    tickling rats 9–10, *10*
    values and reactions 41–42
animal welfare practitioner 1
    animal protection groups 84
    ethologists and veterinarians 84
    ethology 83
    HSUS Farm Animal Welfare 83
    Humane Society International
        colleagues in Vietnam
        82, *83*
    organizations 84
    science-based counterargument 83
anthropomorphizing animals 39
assessment method 52
attitude 21
attitudinal change 21
attribute substitution 38
awareness 37–38

Barbary macaque 61
behavioural intentions *42*
behavioural interaction 3
behavioural prompts 28
Behaviour Change Model 58–59
Behaviour Change Wheel tool 23
Better Chicken 100, **101**
Better Programmes (BPs) 99
broiler chickens 8

camel 118, *119*
Capture–Neuter–Return project *73*
cattle farmers 122–123
cattle feeding 120, *121*
characterizing communities 54–56, **55**
characterizing engagement 56–57, **57**
cognitive biases 38–39
COM-B model 23, 78–79
communitybased enterprises (CBEs) 53
community-based organizations (CBOs) 53
community engagement
    adaptability and localization 52
    adapting strategy *58*
    building on local capacity 52–53
    definitions **49**
    empowerment and ownership 50
    gender roles *51*
    inclusion 50
    levels **57**
    participation 49
    two-way communication 50–52
community leadership 53
confirmation biases 38
corporate social responsibility (CSR) programmes 90
cow protection 126
cultural differences 67
curriculum
    definition 71
    face-to-face format 74
    hidden 71
    online delivery 74
    pedagogical approaches 71–74
    professional requirements 70
customer-driven company 98

Day One veterinary graduate *70*
deficit model 40
digital education 74
donkey 118, *119*

emotional states 2
emotions 41
engagement process 59, *60*, 62
environmental enrichment 37
expert–public gap 40–41
expert *vs.* public 45
external resources 48

farm animal welfare, Nigerian
    African countries 114
    animal welfare practitioner 115–117, *116*
    behavioural change communication 122
    burden/sources 120
    camel 118, *119*
    cattle Farmers 122–123
    cattle feeding 120, *121*
    characteristics 113
    concerns and recommendations 123
    dogs 113
    donkey 118, *119*
    dry season 114
    financial resources 117–118
    funds 117
    good-quality diets 114
    human behaviour 121
    human community 113
    international animal welfare organizations 122
    international NGOs and civil society groups 117
    lack of availability 118
    legal framework 123
    legislation 121
    overcrowded truck 118, *120*
    polo horses 114
    poor animal welfare 118
    pregnant animals 118
    primitive and crude methods 118
    public health issues 122
    rural communities 114
    sick animals 121
    transportation 113–114
farming practices 37
Five Domains Model 98
food businesses 94
food production 82
food supply chains 98
    animal welfare strategy 97–102, 110
    challenges 108–110

corporate sustainability
    professional 103
food business
    agenda 104–105
    commercial animal
        production 104
    larger sustainable agriculture
        space 104
    power of being 105–108
    supplier perspective 105
    IKEA Food 97
    integration 110
formal training 5
frame reflection 44

Global Animal Health (GAH) 161
good environment 3
good health 3
good nutrition 3

habits 28
hands-on teaching/learning 72–73
healthcare system
    animal healthcare providers 165
    global policy or field-level
        interventions 175
    good-quality animal 164, 165
    hard-working horse *164*
    livestock 175
    LMICs 163, 174
    NGO 167
    pain relief medicines, south Africa *173*
    people's livelihoods *166*
    PGCert 162
    problems 167, 168
    relieve pain, East Africa 172–174
    remote settings 166, 167
    veterinary paraprofessional
        mentoring *170*
    welfare appraisal *163*
    welfare livestock programmes,
        Afghanistan 170, 171
    well-functioning animal *162*
    WHO 161
    Working equids, brick kilns of
        Pakistan *169*
    working livestock 165, 166

heuristics 38
hidden curriculum 71
higher-welfare indoor system 8, 12
HSUS Farm Animal Welfare 83
human–animal interaction 28
human behaviour change (HBC) 20
    attitude 21
    education 75, 75–76
    environmental factors 25–26
    fields of research 21, *21*
    habits 28
    intentions 21
    owned 26–27
    principles 28–29, *29*
    process 22–23
    stages 22
    system 27–28
    understanding psychology *see*
        psychology
humane dog population management
    programmes 31
Humane Society International colleagues
    in Vietnam 82, 83
husbandry tools 53
hybrid format 74

India
    active cow shelter 126
    computer-aided dissection 127
    COVID-19 127
    cultural attitudes **128**
    historical worship patterns 126
    livestock production
        management *129*
    Mauryan age 126
    Pashupathi seal' 125
    PCA Act 137, 138
    performing animals
        captive performing
            elephants 135, *136*, 137
        jallikattu bull training 133, 134
        problems 137, 138
    street animals
        cattle 132–134
        dogs 130–132
    Vedic period 125
    vested economic interests 139
    work and life 127–129

information access 37–38
institutional behaviour 78–79
intentions 21
International Coalition for Animal
    Welfare (ICFAW) 84

knowledge translation 36

legislation 121
life-sustaining behaviours 2–3
Low and middle-income countries
    (LMIC) 162

'Madaris' or 'Kalandars' 134
More sustainable animal agriculture
    (MSAA) 97–98
motivation 24–25
Motivational Interviewing (MI) 24

natural habitats, Morocco 61
negative emotional states 2
Non-governmental organizations (NGOs) 82
nutrition campaigns 20

'One Welfare' 1
Organisation for Animal Health (OIE) 2, 163

participatory exercises 32, 32–24, 33
performing animals
    captive performing elephants 135,
        136, 137
    jallikattu bull training 133, 134
    problems 137, 138
Pet Shop Rules (PCA) 138
Planet Positive Strategy (PPP) 97
positive emotional states 3
positive mental experiences 3
postgraduate education 76–77
psychology
    confirmation bias 24
    motivation 24–25
    reactance 24
    social norms 25, 26

public knowledge 37–38
public stakeholders 43–45

quality, definitions of 48–49

rabbits 11–12, *12*
reactance 24
reductionist approach 27
reflective listening 44
resource-poor context
    animal welfare practitioner *see* work
        and life, animal welfare
        practitioner
    donkey toils *142*
    human behaviour change 150–154
    improving NGO 147
    military and police support 141
    problems 149, 150
    welfare appraisal 147, **148**
    working animals 141, 142
        benefits 155, 156
        common welfare issues *149, 150*
Royal Society for the Prevention of
    Cruelty to Animals (RSPCA) 162

science-based advocacy
    animal agriculture 90
    animal behaviour laboratory 88
    animal products 87–88
    animal welfare practitioner *see*
        Animal welfare practitioner
    companies and producers 91
    direct marketing 91, 92
    ethologists/academics 93
    factors 88
    factory farming 82
    farm animal protection movement 90
    farm animal welfare 82, 87
    farmers 94
    food businesses 94
    food production 82
    global progress 92–93
    governments 94
    India 89
    influencers 89
    international supply chains 90

    legal arguments 88
    meat consumption trend 88
    movement grew 82
    multinational companies 90
    public-facing cage- and crate-free
        policies 90
    social justice force 82
    United States 89
    US and European campaigns 91
scientific experts 39–40
social marketing 28
social norms 25, *26*
Society for Applied Ethology (ISAE) 127
strategic engagement 53–54
street animals
    cattle 132–134
    dogs 130–132

Terrestrial Animal Health Code 93
thermal imaging *68*
three spheres framework *36*
tickling rats 9–10, *10*
two-way communication 50–52

United Nations Environment Programme
    (UNEP) 99

veterinary animal welfare education
    68–69, *69*
veterinary practice 22

work and life, animal welfare practitioner
    animal welfare science 144, 145
    Asian elephants 143, *144*
    contextual awareness 145, 146
    development practice 146, 147
    human behaviour 146
    NGO 142
    training/mentoring 147
World Health Organization
    (WHO) 161
World Organisation for Animal Health
    (OIE) 84

zoo welfare workshop 75

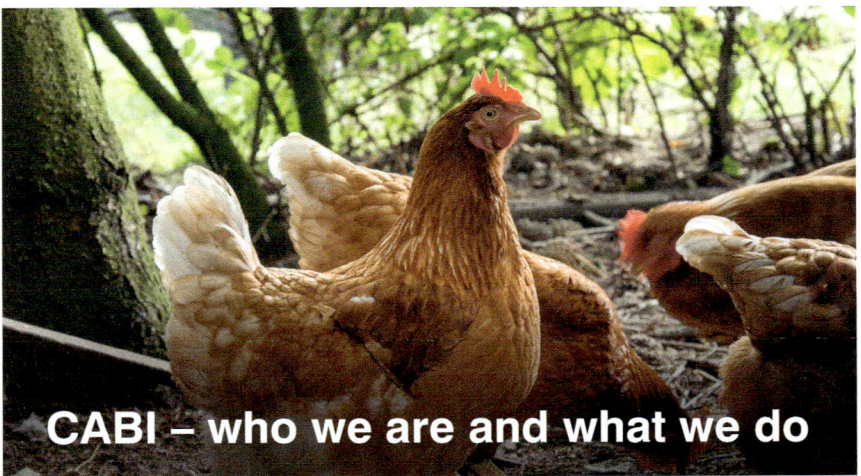

CABI – who we are and what we do

This book is published by **CABI**, an international not-for-profit organisation that improves people's lives worldwide by providing information and applying scientific expertise to solve problems in agriculture and the environment.

CABI is also a global publisher producing key scientific publications, including world renowned databases, as well as compendia, books, ebooks and full text electronic resources. We publish content in a wide range of subject areas including: agriculture and crop science / animal and veterinary sciences / ecology and conservation / environmental science / horticulture and plant sciences / human health, food science and nutrition / international development / leisure and tourism.

The profits from CABI's publishing activities enable us to work with farming communities around the world, supporting them as they battle with poor soil, invasive species and pests and diseases, to improve their livelihoods and help provide food for an ever growing population.

CABI is an international intergovernmental organisation, and we gratefully acknowledge the core financial support from our member countries (and lead agencies) including:

 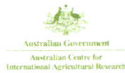 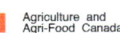 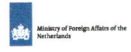 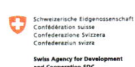

Discover more

To read more about CABI's work, please visit: **www.cabi.org**

Browse our books at: **www.cabi.org/bookshop**,
or explore our online products at: **www.cabi.org/publishing-products**

Interested in writing for CABI? Find our author guidelines here:
www.cabi.org/publishing-products/information-for-authors/